Student Lecture
A Note-Taking Guide to accompany

Discovering Nutrition

Paul Insel
Stanford University

R. Elaine Turner
University of Florida

Don Ross
California Institute of Human Nutrition

Based on the PowerPoint presentation created by
R. Elaine Turner

JONES AND BARTLETT PUBLISHERS
Sudbury, Massachusetts
BOSTON TORONTO LONDON SINGAPORE

World Headquarters
Jones and Bartlett Publishers
40 Tall Pine Drive
Sudbury, MA 01776
978-443-5000
info@jbpub.com
health.jbpub.com

Jones and Bartlett Publishers Canada
2406 Nikanna Road
Mississauga, ON L5C 2W6
CANADA

Jones and Bartlett Publishers International
Barb House, Barb Mews
London W6 7PA
UK

Copyright © 2003 by Jones and Bartlett Publishers, Inc.

All rights reserved. No part of the material protected by this copyright may be reproduced or utilized in any form, electronic or mechanical, including photocopying, recording, or by any information storage and retrieval system, without written permission from the copyright owner.

ISBN: 0-7637-2191-3

Printed in the United States of America
06 05 04   10 9 8 7 6 5 4 3

Contents

How This Book Can Help You Learn Nutrition   v
Note-Taking Tips   vi

Chapter 1   Food Choices: Nutrients and Nourishment   1

Chapter 2   Nutrition Guidelines: Tools for a Healthful Diet   7

Chapter 3   Complementary Nutrition: Functional Foods and Dietary Supplements   13

Chapter 4   The Human Body: From Food to Fuel   17

Chapter 5   Carbohydrates: Simple Sugars and Complex Chains   23

Chapter 6   Lipids: Not Just Fat   29

Chapter 7   Proteins and Amino Acids: Function Follows Form   35

Spotlight on Metabolism   41

Chapter 8   Energy Balance and Weight Management: Finding Your Equilibrium   47

Chapter 9   Vitamins: Vital Keys to Health   51

Spotlight on Alcohol   57

Chapter 10   Water and Minerals: The Ocean Within   61

Chapter 11   Sports Nutrition: Eating for Peak Performance   67

Spotlight on Eating Disorders   73

Chapter 12   Life Cycle: Maternal and Infant Nutrition   77

Chapter 13   Life Cycle: From Childhood through Adulthood   83

Chapter 14   Food Safety and Technology: Microbial Threats and Genetic Engineering   89

Chapter 15   World View of Nutrition: The Faces of Global Malnutrition   93

How This Book Can Help You Learn Nutrition

All of us have different learning styles. Some of us are visual learners, some more auditory, some learn better by doing an activity. Some students prefer to learn new material using visual aids. Some learn material better when they hear it in a lecture; others learn it better by reading it. Cognitive research has shown that no matter what your learning style, you will learn more if you are actively engaged in the learning process.

The Student Lecture Companion will help you learn by providing a structure to your notes and letting you utilize all of the learning styles mentioned above. Students don't need to copy down every word their professor says or recopy their entire textbook. Do the assigned reading, listen in lecture, follow the key points your instructor is making, and write down meaningful notes. After reading and lectures, review your notes and pull out the most important points.

The Student Lecture Companion is your partner and guide in note-taking. Your Companion provides you with a visual guide that follows the chapter topics presented in your textbook, *Discovering Nutrition*. The main topics covered in the lectures are listed in the Table of Contents. No more skimming through chapter after chapter trying to find the term you need to clarify! If your instructor is using the PowerPoint slides that accompany the text, this guide will save you from having to write down everything that is on the slides. There is space provided for you to jot down the terms and concepts that you feel are most important to each lecture. By working with your Companion, you are seeing, hearing, writing, and, later, reading and reviewing. The more times you are exposed to the material, the better you will learn and understand it. Using different methods of exposure significantly increases your comprehension.

Your Companion is the perfect place to write down questions that you want to ask your professor later, interesting ideas that you want to discuss with your study group, or reminders to yourself to go back and study a certain concept again to make sure that you really got it.

Having organized notes is essential at exam time or when doing homework assignments. Your ability to easily locate the important concepts of a recent lecture will help you move along more rapidly, as you don't have to spend time rereading an entire chapter just to reinforce one point that you may not have quite understood.

Your Companion is a valuable resource. You've found a wonderful study partner!

Note-Taking Tips

1. It is easier to take notes if you are not hearing the information for the first time. Read the chapter or the material that is about to be discussed before class. This will help you to anticipate what will be said in class, and have an idea of what to write down. It will also help to read over your notes from the last class. This way you can avoid having to spend the first few minutes of class trying to remember where you left off last time.

2. Don't waste your time trying to write down everything that your professor says. Instead, listen closely and write down only the important points. Review these important points after class to help remind you of related points that were made during the lecture.

3. If the class discussion takes a spontaneous turn, pay attention and participate in the discussion. Only take notes on the conclusions that are relevant to the lecture.

4. Emphasize main points in your notes. You may want to use a highlighter, special notation (asterisks, exclamation points), format (circle, underline), or placement on the page (indented, bulleted). You will find that when you try to recall these points, you will be able to actually picture them on the page.

5. Hearing something repeated, stressed, or summed up can be a signal that it is an important concept to understand.

6. Organize handouts, study guides, and exams in your notebook along with your lecture notes. It may be helpful to use a three-ring binder, so that you can insert pages wherever you need to.

7. When taking notes, you might find it helpful to leave a wide margin on all four sides of the page. Doing this allows you to note names, dates, definitions, etc. for easy access and studying later. It may also be helpful to make notes of questions you want to ask your professor about or research later, ideas or relationships that you want explore more on your own, or concepts that you don't fully understand.

8. It is best to maintain a separate notebook for each class. Labeling and dating your notes can be helpful when you need to look up information from previous lectures.

9. Make your notes legible, and take notes directly in your notebook. Chances are you won't recopy them no matter how noble your intentions. Spend the time you would have spent recopying the notes studying them instead, drawing conclusions and making connections that you didn't have time for in class.

10. Look over your notes after class while the lecture is still fresh in your mind. Fix illegible items and clarify anything you don't understand. Do this again right before the next class.

Chapter 1: Food Choices: Nutrients and Nourishment

Notes

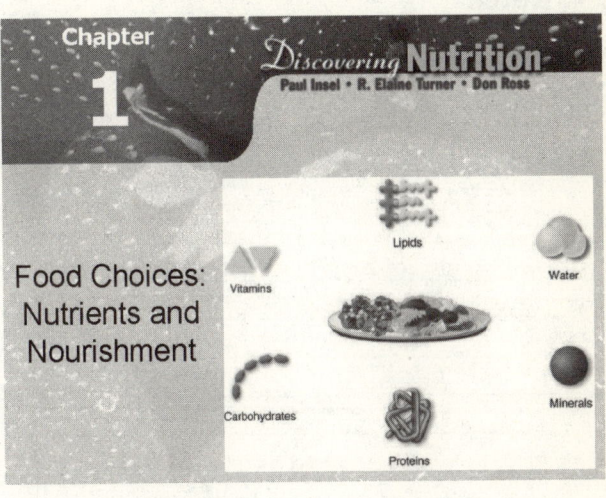

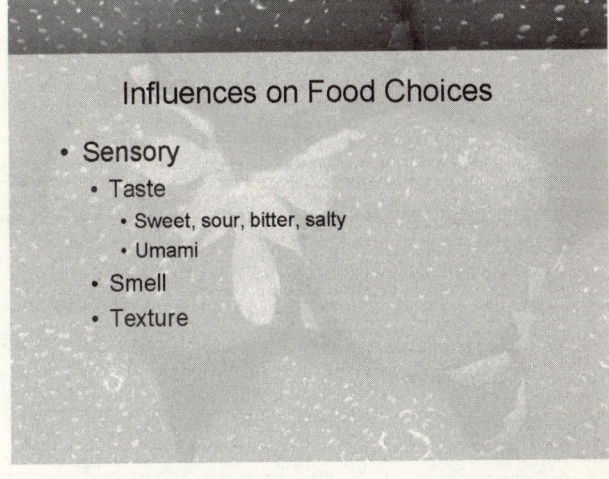

Influences on Food Choices

- Sensory
  - Taste
    - Sweet, sour, bitter, salty
    - Umami
  - Smell
  - Texture

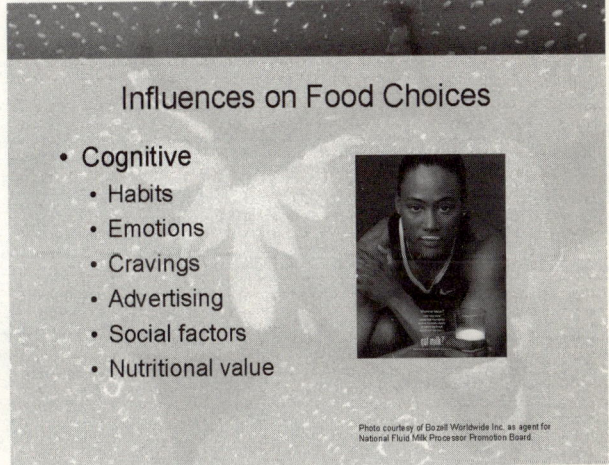

Influences on Food Choices

- Cognitive
  - Habits
  - Emotions
  - Cravings
  - Advertising
  - Social factors
  - Nutritional value

Notes

Influences on Food Choices

- Culture
  - Beliefs and traditions
  - Religion
  - "American diet"

Introducing the Nutrients

- Definition of nutrients
  - Food = mixture of chemicals
  - Essential chemicals = nutrients
  - 6 classes of nutrients
    - Carbohydrates
    - Lipids (fats and oils)
    - Proteins
    - Vitamins
    - Minerals
    - Water

Introducing the Nutrients

- General functions of nutrients
  - Supply energy
    - Carbohydrates, lipids, proteins
  - Contribute to cell and body structure
  - Regulate body processes

Notes

Introducing the Nutrients
- **Carbohydrates**
  - Sugars and starches
  - Functions
    - Energy source
  - Food sources
    - Grains
    - Vegetables
    - Fruits
    - Dairy products

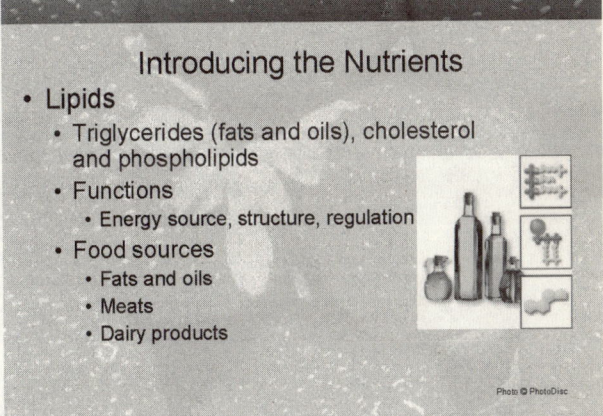

Introducing the Nutrients
- **Lipids**
  - Triglycerides (fats and oils), cholesterol and phospholipids
  - Functions
    - Energy source, structure, regulation
  - Food sources
    - Fats and oils
    - Meats
    - Dairy products

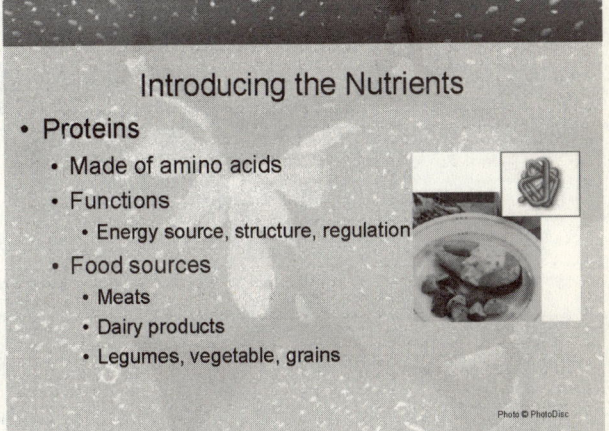

Introducing the Nutrients
- **Proteins**
  - Made of amino acids
  - Functions
    - Energy source, structure, regulation
  - Food sources
    - Meats
    - Dairy products
    - Legumes, vegetable, grains

Notes

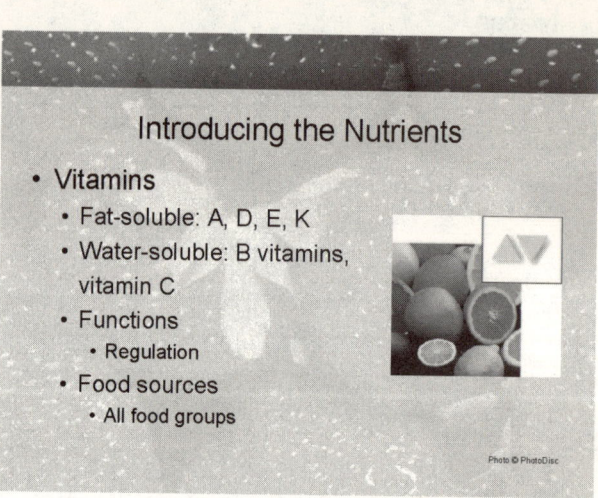

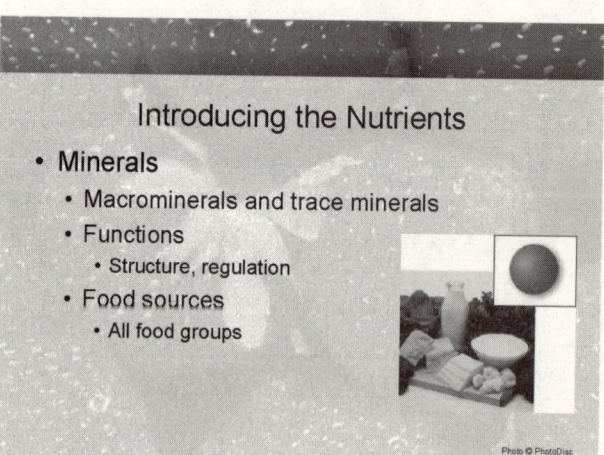

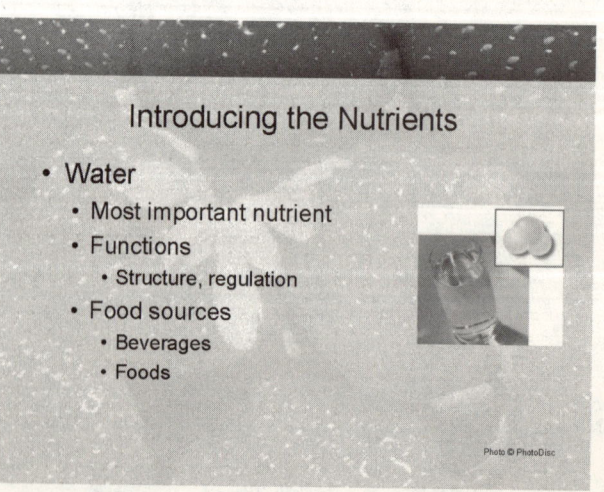

Notes

Introducing the Nutrients

- Energy in foods
  - Measured in kilocalories (kcal)

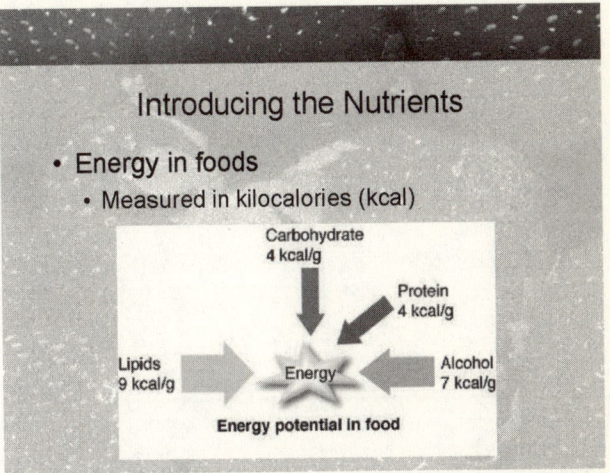

- Carbohydrate 4 kcal/g
- Protein 4 kcal/g
- Lipids 9 kcal/g
- Alcohol 7 kcal/g

Energy potential in food

Applying the Scientific Process to Nutrition

- Scientific method (see Figure 1.11, p. 20)
- Types of studies
  - Epidemiological
  - Animal
  - Cell culture
  - Human
    - Case control
    - Clinical trial

Food Choices: Nutrients and Nourishment

Chapter 2: Nutrition Guidelines: Tools for a Healthful Diet

Notes

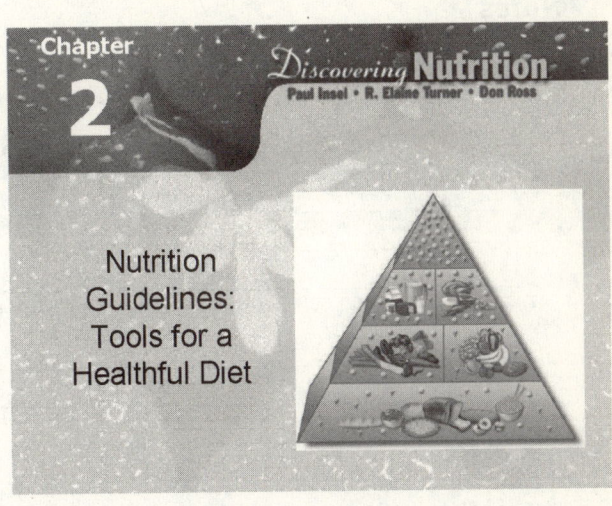

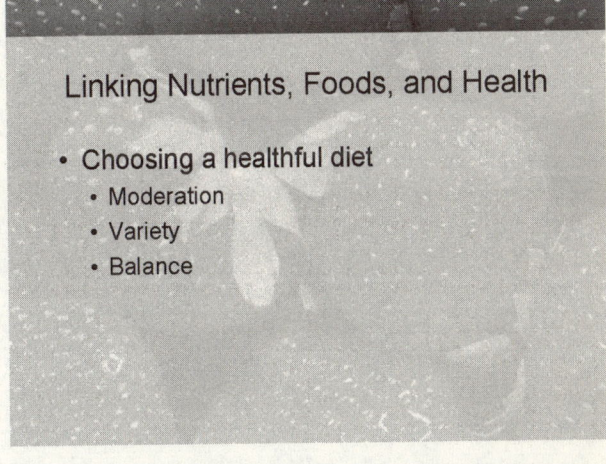

Linking Nutrients, Foods, and Health

- Choosing a healthful diet
  - Moderation
  - Variety
  - Balance

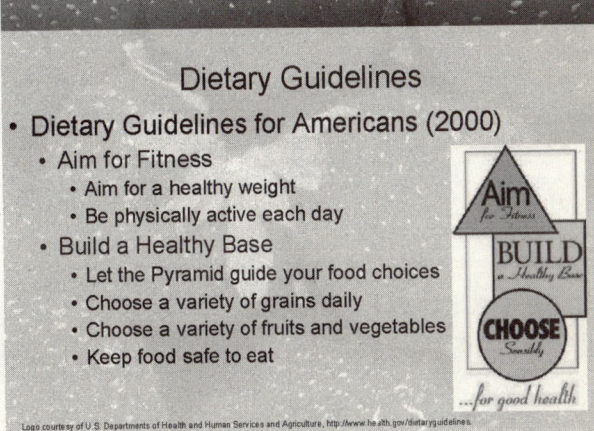

Dietary Guidelines

- Dietary Guidelines for Americans (2000)
  - Aim for Fitness
    - Aim for a healthy weight
    - Be physically active each day
  - Build a Healthy Base
    - Let the Pyramid guide your food choices
    - Choose a variety of grains daily
    - Choose a variety of fruits and vegetables
    - Keep food safe to eat

Notes

Dietary Guidelines

- **Dietary Guidelines for Americans**
  - Choose Sensibly
    - Choose a diet that is low in saturated fat and cholesterol, and moderate in total fat
    - Choose beverages and foods to moderate your intake of sugars
    - Choose and prepare foods with less salt
    - If you drink alcoholic beverages, do so in moderation

Food Groups and Food Guides

- **Food Guide Pyramid**
  - Illustrates many of Dietary Guidelines
  - Food groups
    - Grains: 6-11 servings
    - Vegetables: 3-5 servings
    - Fruits: 2-4 servings
    - Dairy foods: 2-3 servings
    - Meat and alternates: 2-3 servings
    - Fats, oils, and sweets: use sparingly

Food Guide Pyramid

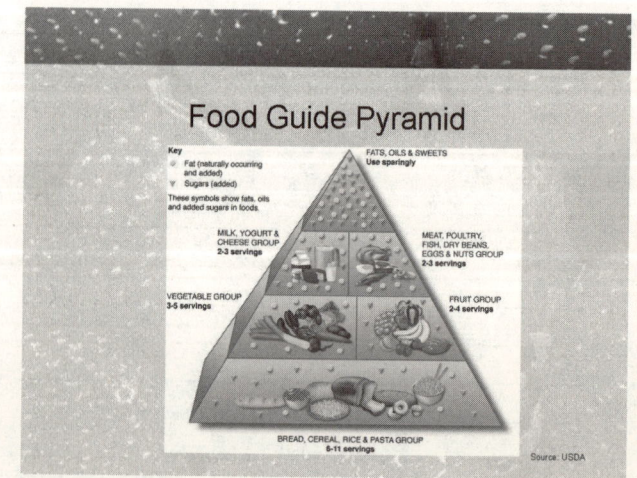

Source: USDA

Notes

Recommendations for Nutrient Intake

- Dietary Reference Intakes (DRIs)
  - Recommendations for nutrient intake
  - Developed by the Food and Nutrition Board
  - Apply to healthy people in the U.S. and Canada
  - Four elements
    - EAR
    - RDA
    - AI
    - UL

Dietary Reference Intakes (DRIs)

- **Estimated Average Requirement (EAR)**
  - Amount that meets the nutrient requirements of 50% of people in a life stage/gender group
  - Based on functional indicator of optimal health
- **Recommended Dietary Allowance**
  - Amount that meets the needs of most people in a life state/gender group

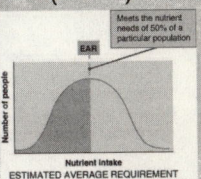
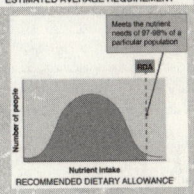

Dietary Reference Intakes (DRIs)

- **Adequate Intake (AI)**
  - Amount thought to be adequate for most people
  - AI used when EAR and RDA can't be determined
- **Tolerable Upper Intake Level (UL)**
  - Intake above the UL can be harmful

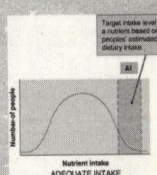
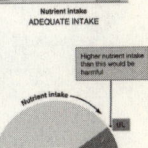

Nutrition Guidelines: Tools for a Healthful Diet

Notes

Dietary Reference Intakes (DRIs)

- Using the DRIs
  - Population groups
    - Assess adequacy of intake
    - Plan diets
    - Set policy and guidelines
  - Individuals
    - Use RDA and AI as target levels for intake
    - Avoid intake > UL

Food Labels

- Mandatory information on food labels
  - Statement of identity
  - Net contents of the package
  - Name and address of manufacturer, packer, distributor
  - List of ingredients
    - Listed in descending order by weight
  - Nutrition information

Food Labels

- Nutrition Facts Panel – standard format

Notes

Food Labels

- Daily Values
  - Compare amount in 1 serving to amount recommended for daily consumption
- Nutrient content claims
  - Descriptive terms, e.g., low fat, high fiber
  - Defined by FDA (see pages 50-51)

Food Labels

- Health claims
  - Link one or more dietary components to reduced risk of disease
  - Must be supported by scientific evidence
  - Approved by FDA (see pages 51-52)
- Structure/Function claims
  - Describe potential effects on body structure or function

Chapter 3: Complementary Nutrition: Functional Foods and Dietary Supplements

Notes

Complementary Nutrition: Functional Foods and Dietary Supplements

Functional Foods

- Provide health benefits beyond nutrition
- Phytochemicals
  - Antioxidants
    - Neutralize free radicals
    - Reduce heart disease, cancer risk
- Found in fruits, vegetables, whole grains, legumes, wine

Food Additives

- Purpose of additives
  - Maintain product consistency
  - Improve nutritional value
  - Maintain quality
  - Provide leavening
  - Enhance flavor or color
- Regulated by FDA
- Subject to Delaney clause

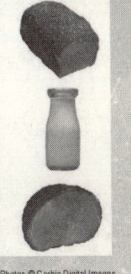

Notes

Dietary Supplements: Vitamins and Minerals

- Moderate supplementation
  - Increased nutrient needs and/or poor intake
    - Pregnant and breastfeeding women
    - Women with heavy menstrual losses
    - Children
    - Infants
    - People with severe food restrictions
    - Strict vegetarians
    - Elders
- No more than 150% of DV

Rational range for vitamin and mineral supplementation: 50% DV – 150% DV (Daily value)

Dietary Supplements: Vitamins and Minerals

- Megadoses
  - Conventional medicine
    - Drug interactions
    - Malabsorption syndromes
    - Treatment of deficiencies
    - Drug-like effects
  - Orthomolecular nutrition
    - Proposed for disease prevention
  - Risks: toxicity from large doses

Dietary Supplements: Natural Health Products

- Herbal therapy (phytotherapy)
  - Traditional medical practices
  - Little scientific evidence of efficacy, safety
- Helpful herbs: examples
  - St. John's wort
  - Milk thistle
  - Ginkgo biloba
  - Saw palmetto
  - Cranberry

Notes

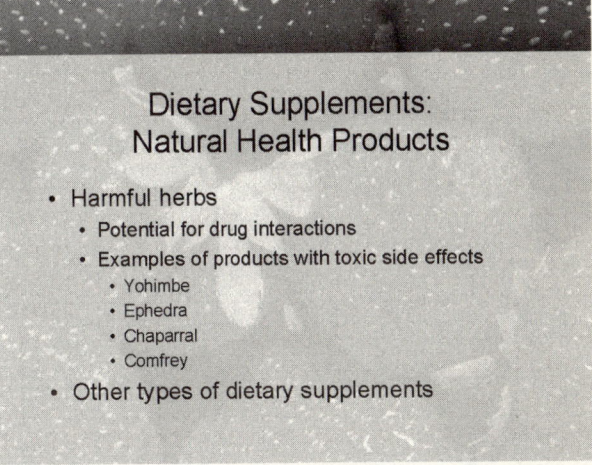

Dietary Supplements: Natural Health Products

- Harmful herbs
  - Potential for drug interactions
  - Examples of products with toxic side effects
    - Yohimbe
    - Ephedra
    - Chaparral
    - Comfrey
- Other types of dietary supplements

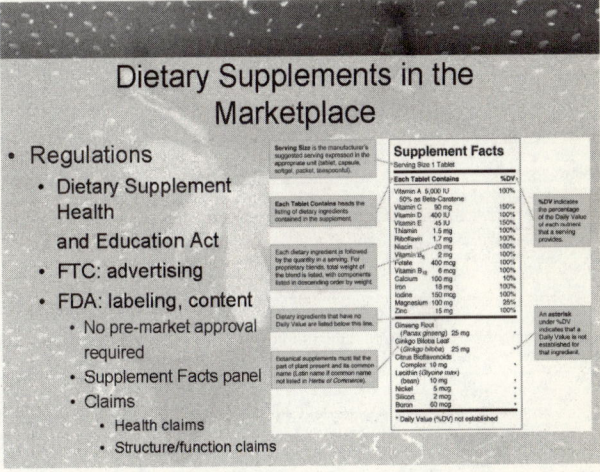

Dietary Supplements in the Marketplace

- Regulations
  - Dietary Supplement Health and Education Act
  - FTC: advertising
  - FDA: labeling, content
    - No pre-market approval required
    - Supplement Facts panel
    - Claims
      - Health claims
      - Structure/function claims

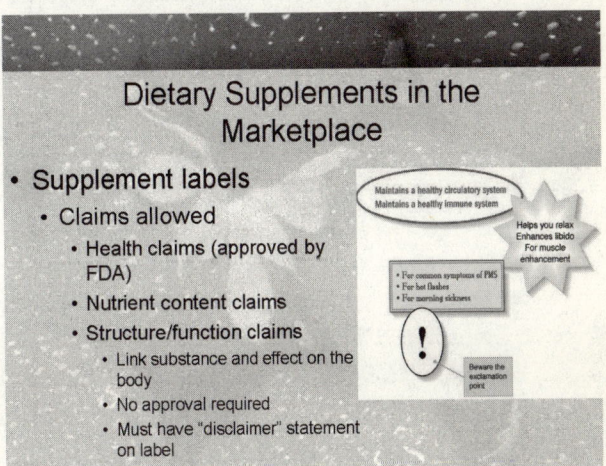

Dietary Supplements in the Marketplace

- Supplement labels
  - Claims allowed
    - Health claims (approved by FDA)
    - Nutrient content claims
    - Structure/function claims
      - Link substance and effect on the body
      - No approval required
      - Must have "disclaimer" statement on label

Complementary Nutrition: Functional Foods and Dietary Supplements

Notes

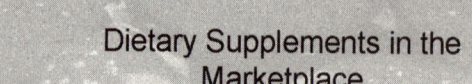

Dietary Supplements in the Marketplace

- Choosing dietary supplements
  - Enough quantity to be effective?
  - How much research has been done?
  - Is it safe?
  - Who is selling the product?
  - Product quality?
- Fraudulent products
  - "too good to be true"

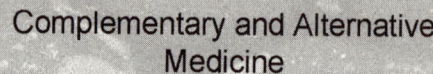

Complementary and Alternative Medicine

- Complementary
  - Practices used in addition to conventional medicine
- Alternative
  - Practices used in place of conventional medicine

Complementary and Alternative Medicine

- Nutrition in CAM
  - Vegetarian diets
  - Macrobiotic diet
  - Food restrictions and prescriptions
  - Need for scientific evaluation

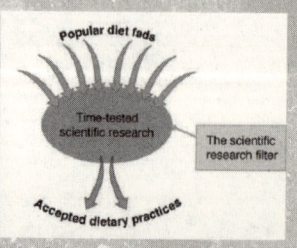

Chapter 4: The Human Body: From Food to Fuel

Notes

The Human Body: From Food to Fuel

The Gastrointestinal Tract

- Organization
  - Mouth → anus
  - Accessory organs
    - Salivary glands, liver, pancreas, gallbladder
- Functions
  - Ingestion
  - Transport
  - Secretion
  - Digestion
  - Absorption
  - Elimination

Overview of Digestion

- Physical movement
  - Peristalsis
  - Segmentation
- Chemical breakdown
  - Enzymes
  - Other secretions

Notes

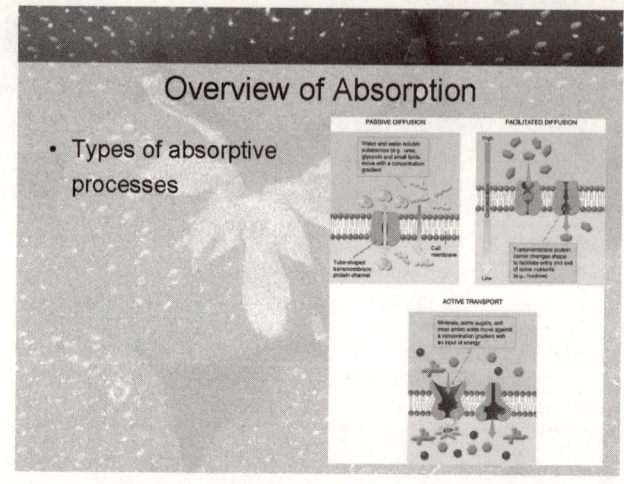

Overview of Absorption

- Types of absorptive processes

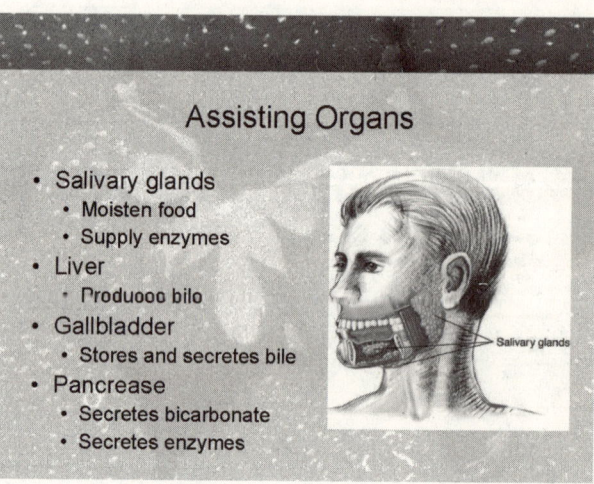

Assisting Organs

- Salivary glands
  - Moisten food
  - Supply enzymes
- Liver
  - Produces bile
- Gallbladder
  - Stores and secretes bile
- Pancrease
  - Secretes bicarbonate
  - Secretes enzymes

Putting It All Together: Digestion and Absorption

- Mouth
  - Enzymes
    - Salivary amylase acts on starch
    - Lingual lipase acts on fat
  - Saliva
    - Moistens food for swallowing
- Esophagus
  - Transports food to stomach
  - Esophageal sphincter

Notes

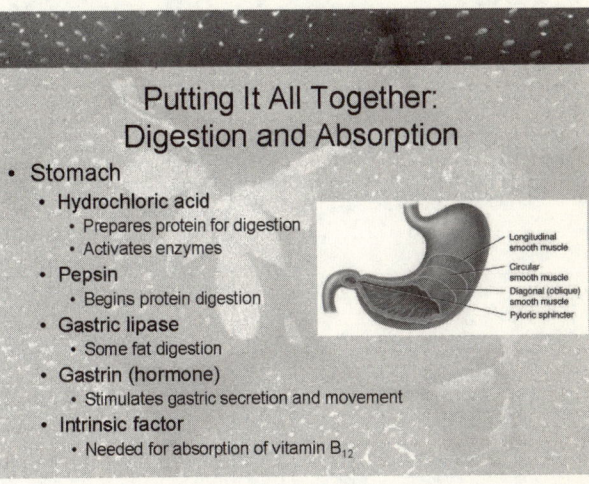

Putting It All Together: Digestion and Absorption

- Stomach
  - Hydrochloric acid
    - Prepares protein for digestion
    - Activates enzymes
  - Pepsin
    - Begins protein digestion
  - Gastric lipase
    - Some fat digestion
  - Gastrin (hormone)
    - Stimulates gastric secretion and movement
  - Intrinsic factor
    - Needed for absorption of vitamin B_{12}

Putting It All Together: Digestion and Absorption

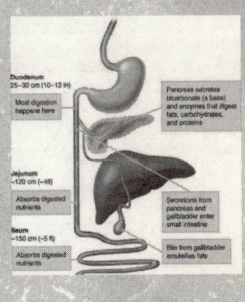

- Small intestine
  - Sections of small intestine
    - Duodenum, jejunum, ileum
  - Digestion
    - Bicarbonate neutralizes stomach acid
    - Pancreatic & intestinal enzymes
      - Carbohydrates
      - Fat
      - Protein

Putting It All Together: Digestion and Absorption

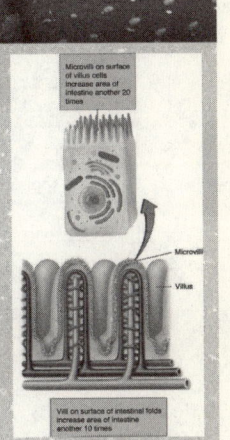

- Small intestine
  - Absorption
    - Folds, villi, microvilli expand absorptive surface
    - Most nutrients absorbed here
    - Fat-soluble nutrients go into lymph
    - Other nutrients into blood

The Human Body: From Food to Fuel

Notes

Putting It All Together: Digestion and Absorption

- Large Intestine
  - Digestion
    - Nutrient digestion already complete
    - Some digestion of fiber by bacteria
  - Absorption
    - Water
    - Sodium, potassium, chloride
    - Vitamin K (produced by bacteria)
  - Elimination

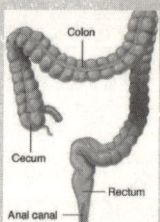

Circulation of Nutrients

- Vascular system
- Lymphatic system
- Excretion and elimination

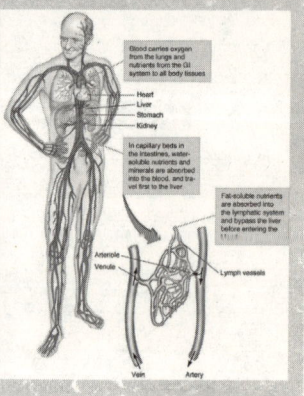

Signaling Systems: Command, Control, Defense

- Nervous system
  - Regulates GI activity
    - Local system of nerves
    - Central nervous system
- Hormonal system
  - Increases or decreases GI activity
- Immune system
  - Identifies and attacks foreign invaders

Notes

Nutrition and GI Disorders

- Constipation
  - Hard, dry, infrequent stools
  - Reduced by high fiber, fluid intake, exercise
- Diarrhea
  - Loose, watery, frequent stools
  - Symptom of diseases/infections
  - Can cause dehydration
- Diverticulosis
  - Pouches along colon
  - High fiber diet reduces formation

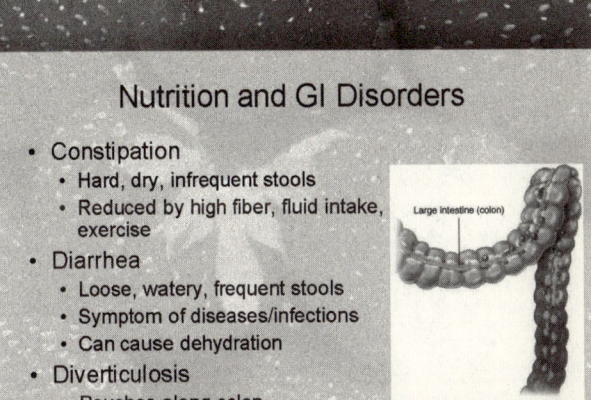

Nutrition and GI Disorders

- Gastroesophageal Reflux Disease (GERD)
  - Reduced by smaller meals, less fat
- Irritable Bowel Syndrome (IBS)
- Colon cancer
  - Antioxidants may reduce risk
- Gas
- Ulcers
  - Bacterial cause
- Functional dyspepsia

Chapter 5: Carbohydrates: Simple Sugars and Complex Chains

Notes

Carbohydrates

- Sugars, Starches, Fibers
- Major food sources: plants
  - Formed during photosynthesis

Simple Sugars: Monosaccharides and Disaccharides

- Monosaccharides – single sugar unit
  - Glucose
    - Found in fruits, vegetables, honey
    - "blood sugar" – used for energy
  - Fructose
    - "fruit sugar"
    - Found in fruits, honey, corn syrup
  - Galactose
    - Found as part of lactose in milk

Simple Sugars: Monosaccharides and Disaccharides

- Disaccharides – two linked sugar units
  - Sucrose: glucose + fructose
    - "table sugar"
    - Made from sugar cane and sugar beets
  - Lactose: glucose + galactose
    - "milk sugar"
    - Found in milk and dairy products
  - Maltose: glucose + glucose
    - Found in germinating cereal grains
    - Product of starch breakdown

Notes

Complex Carbohydrates
- Starch
  - Long chains of glucose units
    - Amylose – straight chains
    - Amylopectin – branched chains
  - Found in grains, vegetables, legumes
- Glycogen
  - Highly branched chains of glucose units
  - Body's storage form of carbohydrate

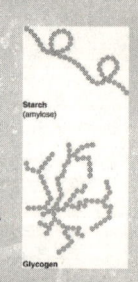

Complex Carbohydrates
- Dietary Fiber
  - Indigestible chains of monosaccharides
    - Oligosaccharides: short chains
    - Non-starch polysaccharides: long chains
      - Cellulose, hemicellulose, pectins, gums, mucilages
    - Lignins
  - Found in fruits, vegetables, grains, legumes

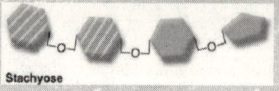
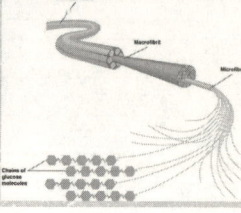

Carbohydrate Digestion and Absorption
- Mouth
  - Salivary amylase begins digestion of starch
- Small intestine
  - Pancreatic amylase completes starch digestion
  - Brush border enzymes digest disaccharides
- End products of carbohydrate digestion
  - Glucose, fructose, galactose
  - Absorbed into bloodstream
- Fibers are not digested, excreted in feces

Notes

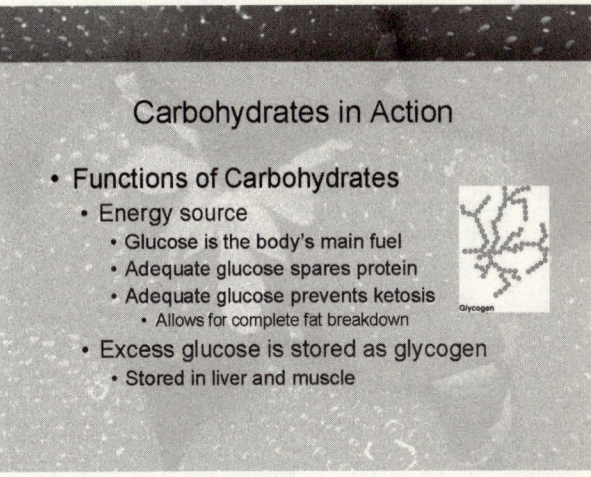

Carbohydrates in Action

- **Functions of Carbohydrates**
  - Energy source
    - Glucose is the body's main fuel
    - Adequate glucose spares protein
    - Adequate glucose prevents ketosis
      - Allows for complete fat breakdown
  - Excess glucose is stored as glycogen
    - Stored in liver and muscle

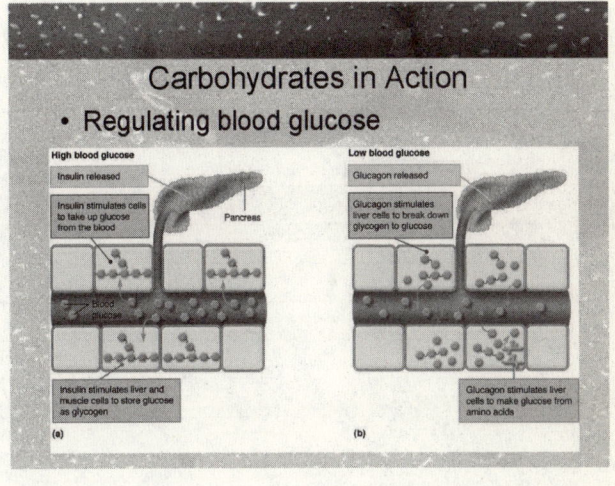

Carbohydrates in Action

- **Regulating blood glucose**

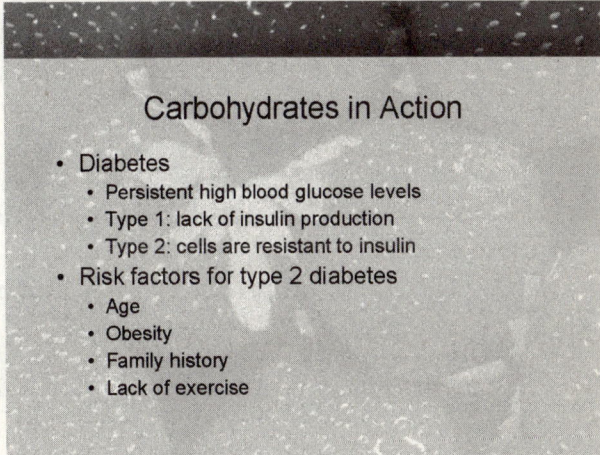

Carbohydrates in Action

- Diabetes
  - Persistent high blood glucose levels
  - Type 1: lack of insulin production
  - Type 2: cells are resistant to insulin
- Risk factors for type 2 diabetes
  - Age
  - Obesity
  - Family history
  - Lack of exercise

Carbohydrates: Simple Sugars and Complex Chains

Notes

Carbohydrates in Your Diet

- Recommended carbohydrate intake
  - 55-60% of kilocalories
  - Daily Value (for 2,000 kcal) = 300 grams
  - Dietary Guidelines
    - Moderate sugar intake
    - Variety of grains, fruits, vegetables

Carbohydrates in Your Diet

- Increasing complex carbohydrate intake
  - Grains, especially whole grains
  - Legumes
  - Vegetables

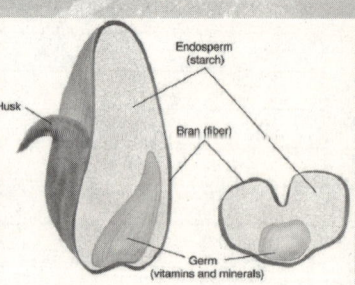

Carbohydrates in Your Diet

- Reducing sugar intake
  - Use less added sugar
  - Limit soft drinks, sugary cereals, candy
  - Choose fresh fruits or those canned in water or juice

Notes

Carbohydrates in Your Diet

- Artificial Sweeteners
  - Minimal or zero kcal
  - Many times sweeter than sugar
  - Non-cariogenic (don't promote tooth decay)
  - Current products
    - Saccharin
    - Aspartame
    - Acesulfame
    - Sucralose
- Sugar alcohols
  - ~2 kcal/gram
  - Non-cariogenic

Carbohydrates and Health

- High sugar intake
  - Low nutrient content
  - Contributes to tooth decay
  - If excess kcal, contributes to obesity
- High fiber intake
  - Better control of blood glucose
  - Possible reduced cancer risk
  - Reduced risk of heart disease
  - Healthier gastrointestinal functioning

Chapter 6: Lipids: Not Just Fat

Notes

Lipids

- Triglycerides
- Phospholipids
- Sterols

Fatty Acids are Key Building Blocks

- Types of fatty acids
  - Saturated
    - All single bonds between carbons
  - Monounsaturated
    - One carbon-carbon double bond
  - Polyunsaturated
    - More than one carbon-carbon double bond

Fatty Acids Are Key Building Blocks

- Types of fatty acids
  - Cis and trans
    - Hydrogenation produces trans fatty acids
  - Essential fatty acids
    - Linoleic acid and alpha-linolenic acid
    - Can't be made in the body
    - Used to make eicosanoids

Notes

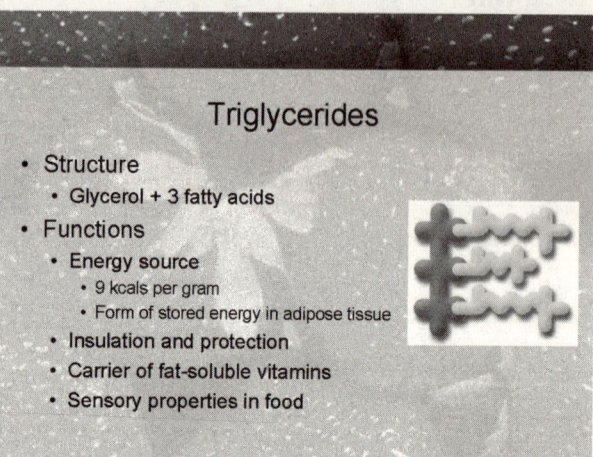

Triglycerides
- Structure
  - Glycerol + 3 fatty acids
- Functions
  - Energy source
    - 9 kcals per gram
    - Form of stored energy in adipose tissue
  - Insulation and protection
  - Carrier of fat-soluble vitamins
  - Sensory properties in food

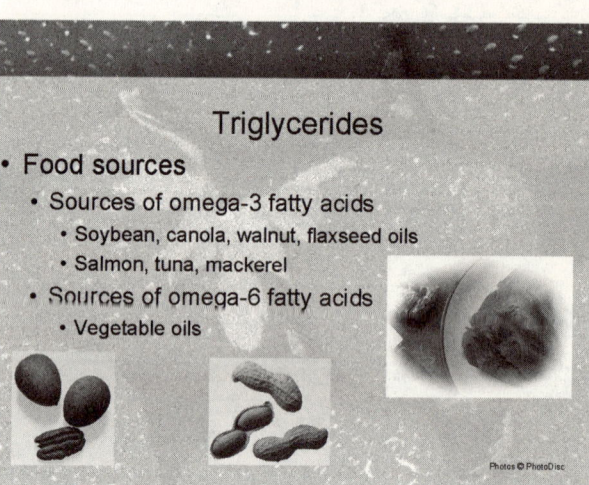

Triglycerides
- Food sources
  - Sources of omega-3 fatty acids
    - Soybean, canola, walnut, flaxseed oils
    - Salmon, tuna, mackerel
  - Sources of omega-6 fatty acids
    - Vegetable oils

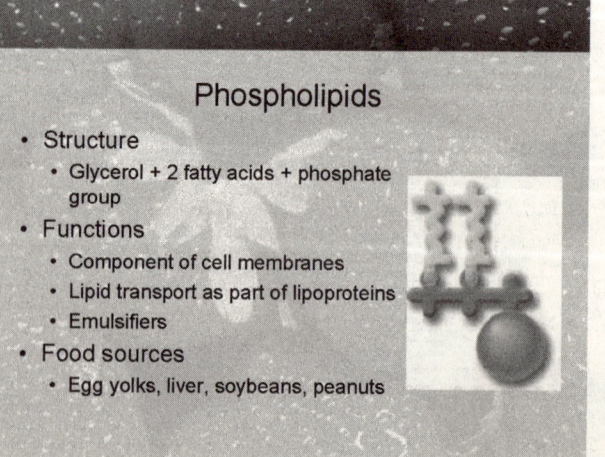

Phospholipids
- Structure
  - Glycerol + 2 fatty acids + phosphate group
- Functions
  - Component of cell membranes
  - Lipid transport as part of lipoproteins
  - Emulsifiers
- Food sources
  - Egg yolks, liver, soybeans, peanuts

Notes

Sterols: Cholesterol

- Functions
  - Component of cell membranes
  - Precursor to other substances
    - Sterol hormones
    - Vitamin D
    - Bile acids
- Synthesis
  - Made mainly in the liver
- Food sources
  - Found only in animal foods

Digestion and Absorption

- Mouth and stomach
  - Minimal digestion of triglycerides
- Small intestine
  - Emulsified by phospholipids
  - Digested by pancreatic lipase
  - Absorbed into intestinal cells
    - Formed into chylomicrons and moved into lymphatic system

Lipids in the Body

- Lipoproteins carry lipids around the body
  - Chylomicrons
    - Delivers dietary lipids from intestines to cells and liver
  - Very-low-density lipoproteine (VLDL)
    - Delivers triglycerides to cells
  - Low-density lipoproteins (LDL)
    - Delivers cholesterol to cells
  - High density lipoproteins (HDL)
    - Picks up cholesterol for removal or recycling

Notes

Lipids in the Diet

- **Recommended intake**
  - Reduce total fat, saturated fat, and cholesterol
  - Need ~ 2% of kcals as essential fatty acids
  - Improve balance of omega-3: omega-6 fatty acids

Lipids in the Diet

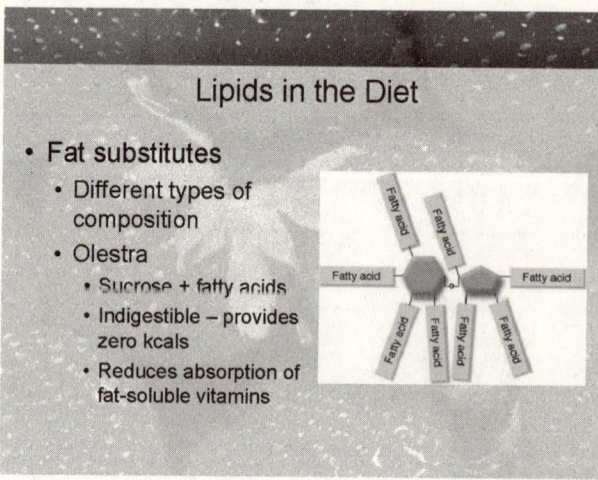

- **Fat substitutes**
  - Different types of composition
  - Olestra
    - Sucrose + fatty acids
    - Indigestible – provides zero kcals
    - Reduces absorption of fat-soluble vitamins

Lipids and Health

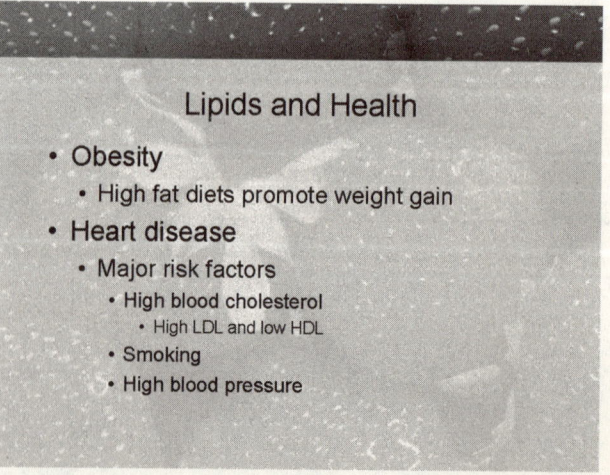

- **Obesity**
  - High fat diets promote weight gain
- **Heart disease**
  - Major risk factors
    - High blood cholesterol
      - High LDL and low HDL
    - Smoking
    - High blood pressure

Notes

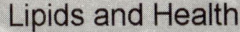

Lipids and Health
- Reducing heart disease risk
  - Lifestyle
    - Stop smoking, increase exercise, manage weight and blood pressure
  - Diet
    - Reduce saturated fat, cholesterol, total fat
    - Increase antioxidants
    - Increase B-vitamins
    - Increase omega-3 fatty acids
    - Increase dietary fiber
    - Other factors

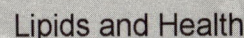

Lipids and Health
- Cancer
  - Stages of development
    - Initiation, promotion, progression
  - Reducing cancer risk
    - Eat a variety of healthful foods; plant sources
    - Be more physically active
    - Maintain a healthful weight
    - Limit alcohol consumption

Chapter 7: Proteins and Amino Acids: Function Follows Form

Notes

Proteins and Amino Acids

Amino Acids Are the Building Blocks of Protein

- Proteins are sequences of amino acids
- Types of amino acids
  - Essential: most come from diet
  - Nonessential: can be made in the body

Amino Acids Are the Building Blocks of Protein

- Protein structure
  - Chain of amino acids
    - Sequence of amino acids determines shape
    - Shape of protein determines function
  - Denaturing protein structure
    - Disrupts function
    - Caused by heat, acid, oxidation, agitation

Notes

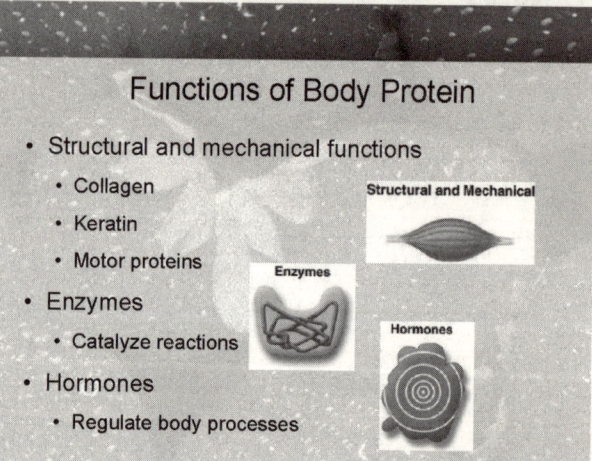

Functions of Body Protein
- Structural and mechanical functions
  - Collagen
  - Keratin
  - Motor proteins
- Enzymes
  - Catalyze reactions
- Hormones
  - Regulate body processes

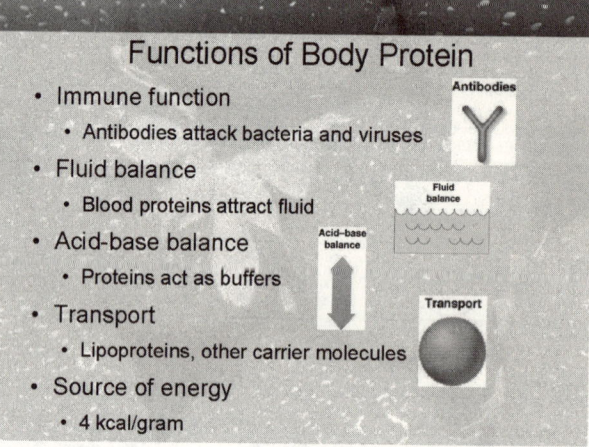

Functions of Body Protein
- Immune function
  - Antibodies attack bacteria and viruses
- Fluid balance
  - Blood proteins attract fluid
- Acid-base balance
  - Proteins act as buffers
- Transport
  - Lipoproteins, other carrier molecules
- Source of energy
  - 4 kcal/gram

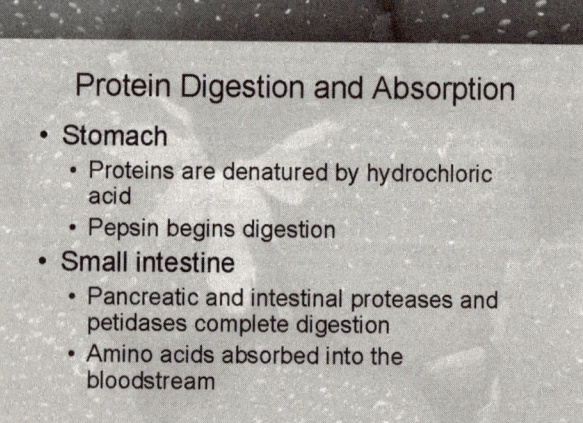

Protein Digestion and Absorption
- Stomach
  - Proteins are denatured by hydrochloric acid
  - Pepsin begins digestion
- Small intestine
  - Pancreatic and intestinal proteases and petidases complete digestion
  - Amino acids absorbed into the bloodstream

Notes

Proteins in the Body
- Protein synthesis
  - Directed by cellular DNA
- Protein excretion
  - Deamination of amino acids
  - Amino groups converted to urea for excretion
- Nitrogen balance
  - Nitrogen intake vs. nitrogen output

Proteins in the Diet
- Recommended protein intake
  - Adult RDA = 0.8 grams/kilogram body weight
  - Infant RDA = 2.2 grams/kilogram body weight
- Increased protein needs
  - Physical stress
  - Injury
  - Intense weight training
- U.S. protein intake > protein needs

Proteins in the Diet
- Protein quality
  - Complete proteins
    - supply all essential amino acids
    - animal proteins, soy proteins
  - Incomplete proteins
    - low in one or more essential amino acids
    - most plant proteins
  - Complementary proteins
    - 2 incomplete proteins = complete protein

Photo courtesy of the USDA

Notes

Proteins in the Diet

- Evaluating protein quality
  - Amino acid composition
  - Digestibility
  - Protein Digestibility-Corrected Amino Acid Score (PDCAAS)
    - Used to determine %DV
- Protein and amino acid supplements
  - Generally not needed
  - Risks unknown

The Pros and Cons of Vegetarian Eating

- Types of vegetarian diets
  - Semi-vegetarian
  - Lacto-ovo vegetarian
  - Vegan
- Health benefits
  - Less fat, saturated fat, cholesterol
    - Reduced heart disease risk
    - Reduced obesity
    - Reduced hypertension
    - Reduced cancer risk

The Pros and Cons of Vegetarian Eating

- Health risks
  - Vegan diets
    - Low in calcium, iron, zinc, vitamin D, vitamin B_{12}, vitamin B_6
  - More restrictive diets – less nutrient adequacy
  - Careful planning to meet needs of children, pregnant women
- Dietary recommendations
  - Variety is important
  - Vegetarian pyramid: Figure 7.13

Notes

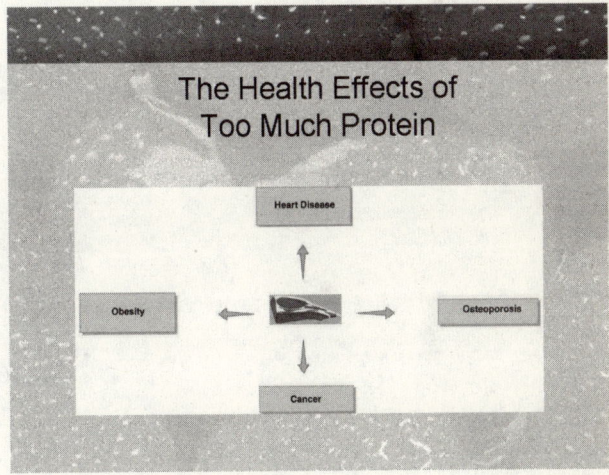

The Health Effects of Too Little Protein

- Protein-Energy malnutrition (PEM)
  - Kwashiorkor
  - Marasmus

The Health Effects of Too Much Protein

- Heart Disease
- Obesity
- Osteoporosis
- Cancer

Proteins and Amino Acids: Function Follows Form

Spotlight on Metabolism

Notes

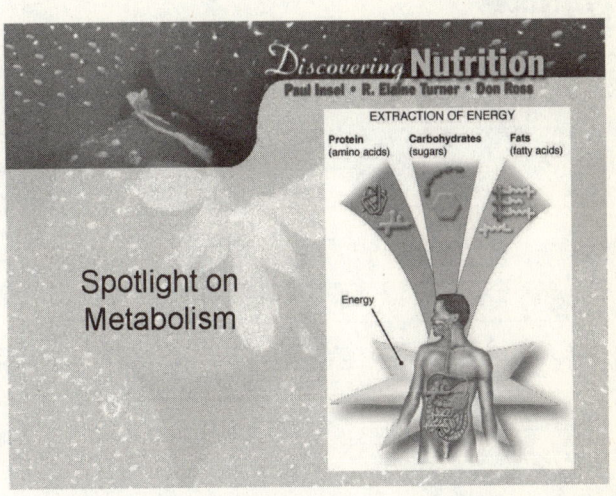

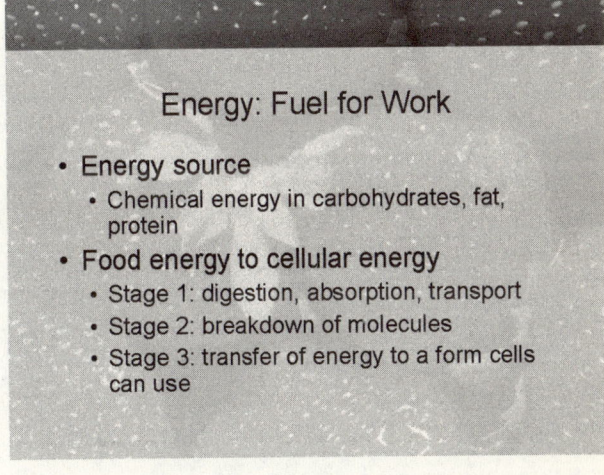

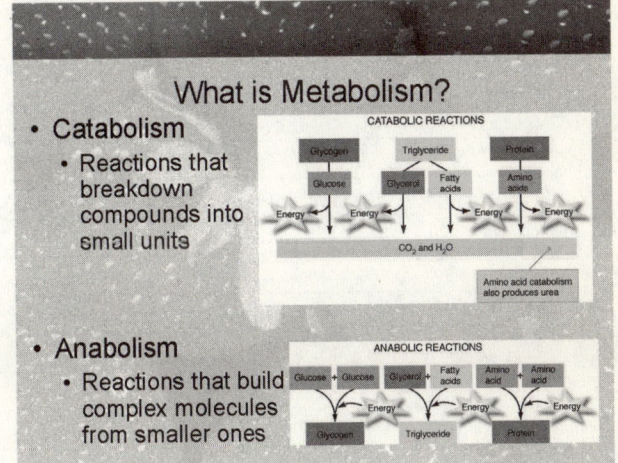

Notes

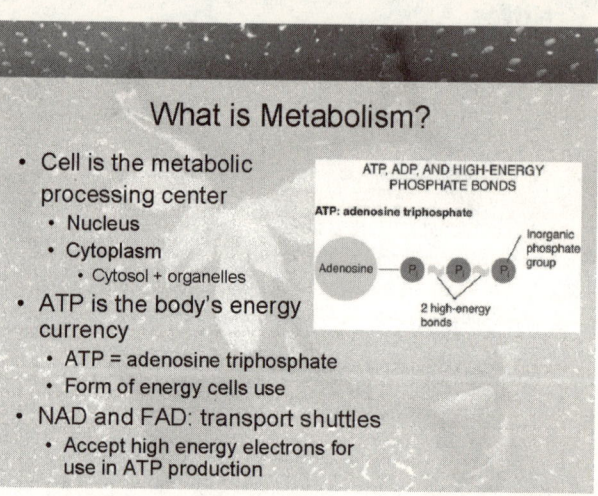

What is Metabolism?
- Cell is the metabolic processing center
  - Nucleus
  - Cytoplasm
    - Cytosol + organelles
- ATP is the body's energy currency
  - ATP = adenosine triphosphate
  - Form of energy cells use
- NAD and FAD: transport shuttles
  - Accept high energy electrons for use in ATP production

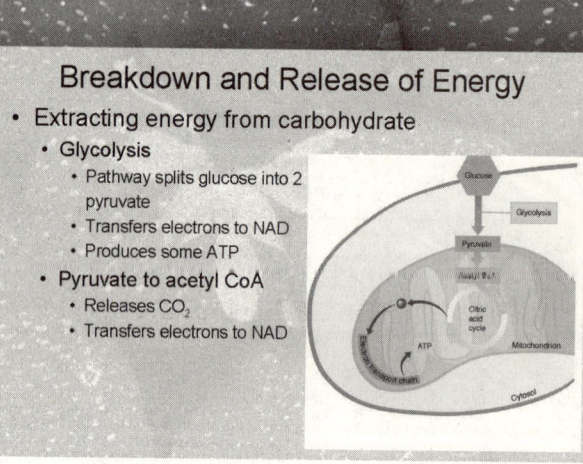

Breakdown and Release of Energy
- Extracting energy from carbohydrate
  - Glycolysis
    - Pathway splits glucose into 2 pyruvate
    - Transfers electrons to NAD
    - Produces some ATP
  - Pyruvate to acetyl CoA
    - Releases CO_2
    - Transfers electrons to NAD

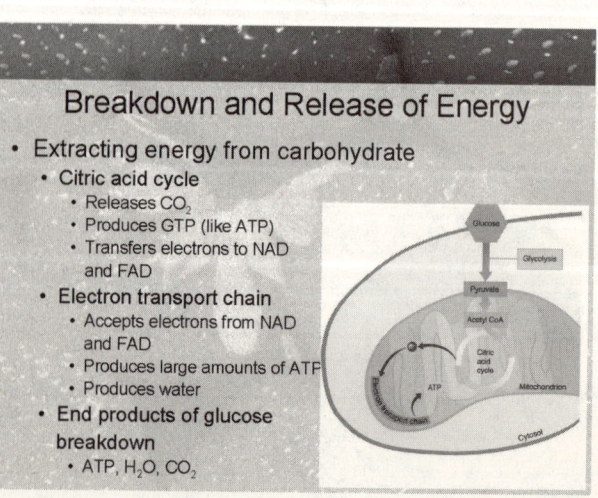

Breakdown and Release of Energy
- Extracting energy from carbohydrate
  - Citric acid cycle
    - Releases CO_2
    - Produces GTP (like ATP)
    - Transfers electrons to NAD and FAD
  - Electron transport chain
    - Accepts electrons from NAD and FAD
    - Produces large amounts of ATP
    - Produces water
  - End products of glucose breakdown
    - ATP, H_2O, CO_2

Notes

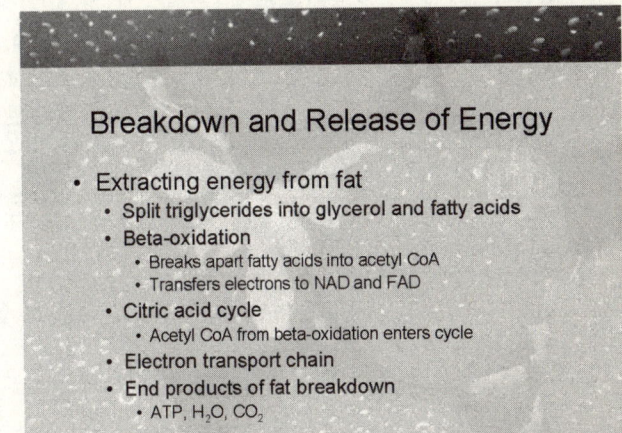

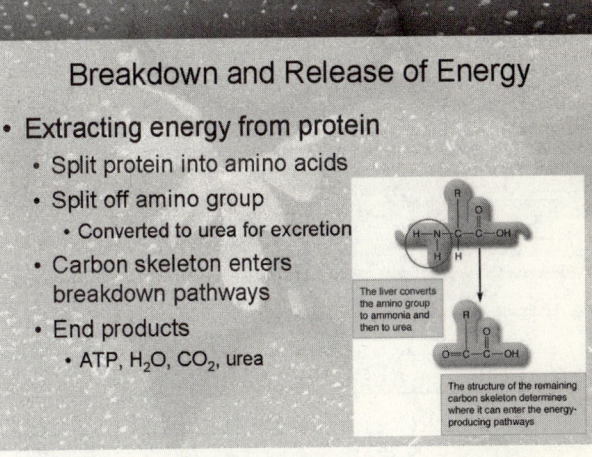

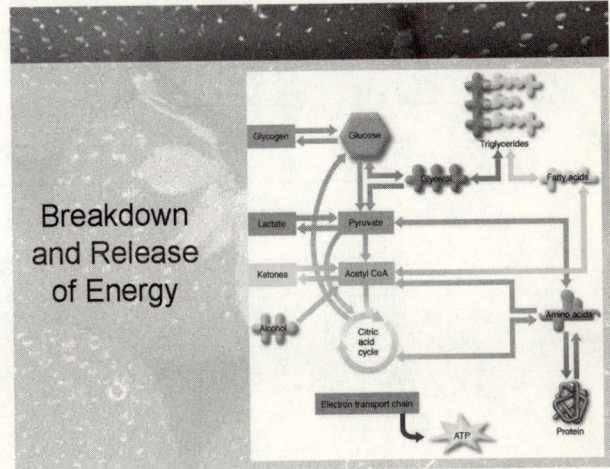

Notes

Biosynthesis and Storage

- Making carbohydrate (glucose)
  - Gluconeogenesis
    - Uses pyruvate, lactate, glycerol, certain amino acids
- Storing carbohydrate (glycogen)
  - Liver, muscle make glycogen from glucose
- Making fat (fatty acids)
  - Lipogenesis
    - Uses acetyl CoA from fat, amino acids, glucose
- Storing fat (triglyceride)
  - Stored in adipose tissue

Biosynthesis and Storage

- Making ketone bodies (ketogenesis)
  - Made from acetyl CoA
    - Inadequate glucose in cells
- Making protein (amino acids)
  - Amino acid pool supplied from
    - Diet, protein breakdown, cell synthesis

Special States

- Feasting
  - Excess energy intake from carbohydrate, fat, protein
    - Promotes storage

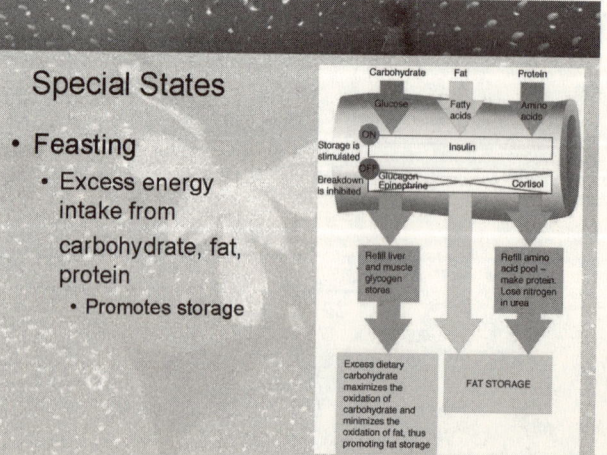

Notes

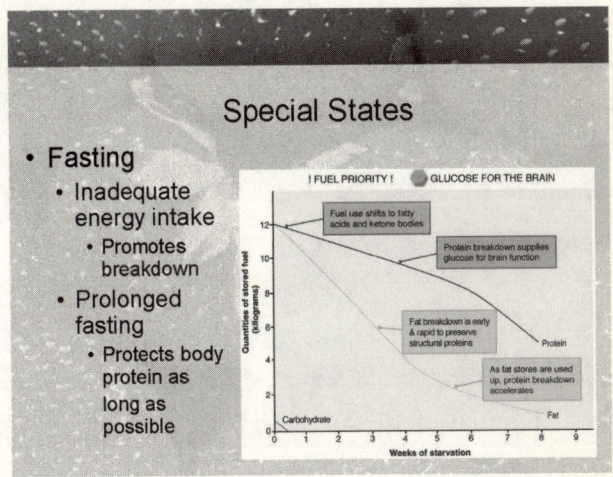

Spotlight on Metabolism

Chapter 8: Energy Balance and Weight Management: Finding Your Equilibrium

Notes

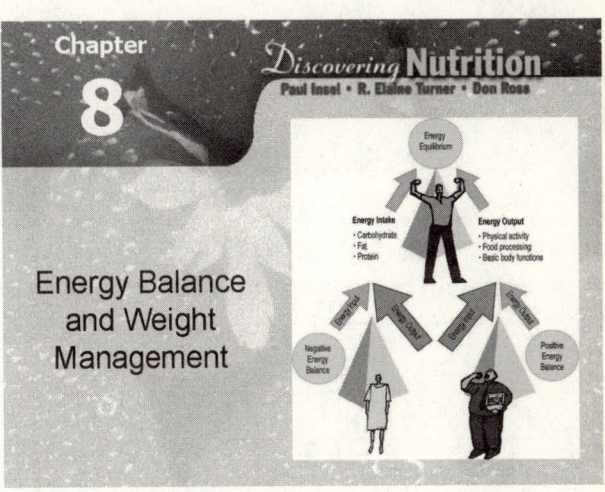

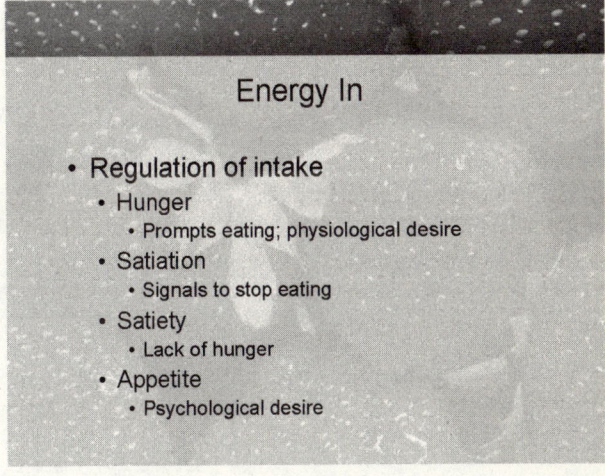

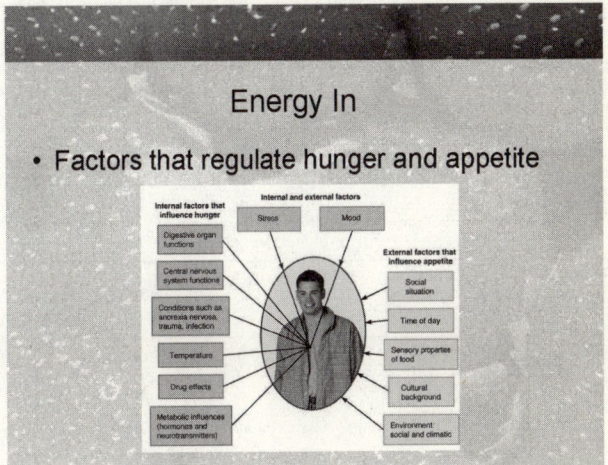

Notes

Energy Out: Fuel Uses
- Major components of energy expenditure
  - Resting energy expenditure (REE)
    - Energy for basic body functions
    - Affected by body size, composition, age, gender
  - Physical activity
    - Highly variable
    - Affected by body size, fitness level, type of activity
  - Thermic effect of food (TEF)
    - Energy to digest, absorb, metabolize food

Thermic effect of food (~10%)
Physical activity (15–30%)
Resting energy expenditure (60–75%)

Body Composition: Understanding Fatness and Weight
- Assessing body weight
  - Height-weight tables
  - Body mass index (BMI)
    - Weight (kg) ÷ height^2 (m)
- Assessing body fatness
- Body fat distribution
  - Waist circumference

When Energy Balance Goes Awry
- Definitions
  - Overweight: BMI between 25-30
  - Obesity: BMI > 30
  - Underweight: BMI < 18.5
- Health risks of overweight and obesity
  - Heart disease and stroke
  - Hypertension
  - Diabetes
  - Cancer
  - Joint diseases

Notes

When Energy Balance Goes Awry

- Early theories of weight regulation
  - Fat cell theory
    - Obesity increases number and size of fat cells
  - Set point theory
- Influences on weight gain and obesity
  - Heredity and genetic factors
  - Sociocultural influences
  - Age and lifestyle factors
  - Gender and ethnicity
  - Socioeconomic factors
  - Psychological factors

Weight Management

- Perception of weight
- Setting realistic goals
- Weight management lifestyle
  - Diet and eating habits
    - Reduce total calories
    - Reduce fat calories
    - Increase complex carbohydrates
    - Improve eating habits
- Increase physical activity
- Stress management
- Self-acceptance

Weight Management

- Weight management approaches
  - Self-help books and manuals
    - Watch for signs of a fad diet
  - Self-help groups
  - Commercial programs
  - Professional counselors
  - Prescription drugs
  - OTC drugs and dietary supplements

Energy Balance and Weight Management: Finding Your Equilibrium

Notes

Weight Management

- Weight management approaches
  - Surgery

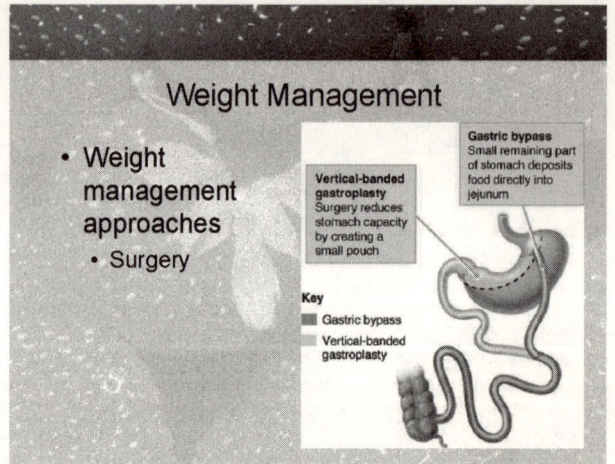

Underweight

- Definition
  - BMI < 18.5
- Causes and assessment
  - Illness
  - Eating disorders
  - Metabolic factors
- Weight-gain strategies
  - Small, frequent meals
  - Fluids between meals
  - High-calorie foods and beverages

Chapter 9: Vitamins: Vital Keys to Health

Notes

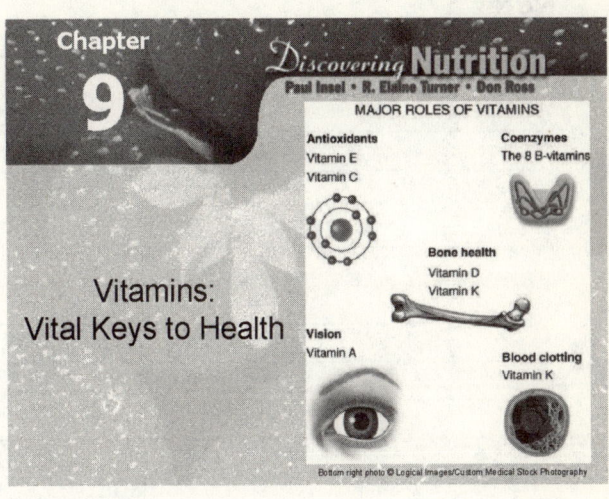

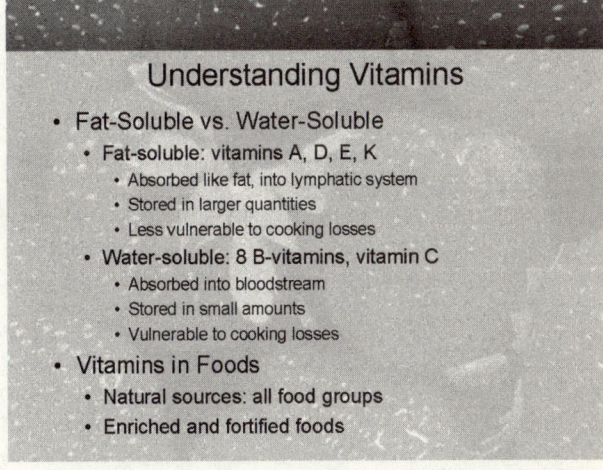

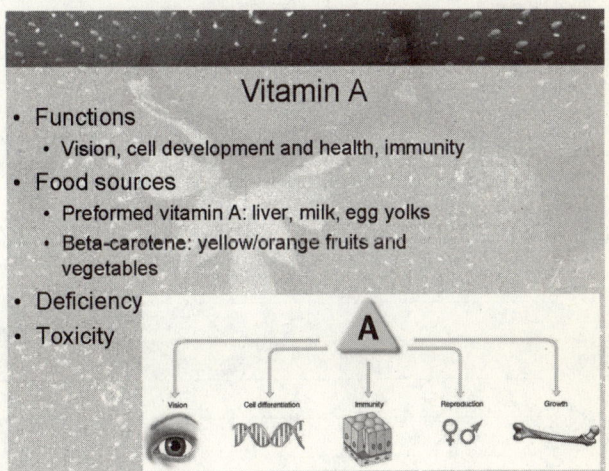

Notes

Vitamin D
- Synthesis
  - Made in the skin from cholesterol
  - Activated in liver and kidney
- Functions
  - Regulates blood calcium levels
- Food sources
  - Fortified milk, fortified cereals
- Deficiency
  - Rickets in children; osteomalacia in adults
- Toxicity

Vitamin E
- Functions
  - Antioxidant
- Food Sources
  - Nuts and seeds
  - Wheat germ
  - Oils, margarine, salad dressing
- Deficiency
- Toxicity

Vitamin K
- Functions
  - Blood clotting
  - Formation of bone
- Food sources
  - Green vegetables, liver, egg yolks
- Deficiency
- Interferes with anticoagulant medications

Notes

Thiamin
- Functions
  - Coenzyme in energy metabolism
  - Helps synthesize neurotransmitters
- Food sources
  - Whole and enriched grains
  - Pork, legumes, seeds, nuts, liver
- Deficiency
  - Beriberi

Riboflavin
- Functions
  - Coenzyme in energy metabolism
  - Supports antioxidants
- Food sources
  - Milk and dairy products
  - Whole and enriched grains
- Deficiency
  - ariboflavinosis

Niacin
- Functions
  - Coenzyme in energy metabolism
  - Supports fatty acid synthesis
- Food sources
  - Whole and enriched grains
  - Meat, poultry, fish, nuts, and peanuts
- Deficiency
  - pellagra
- Toxicity
  - High doses used to treat high blood cholesterol
  - Side effects: skin flushing, liver damage

Vitamins: Vital Keys to Health

Notes

Vitamin B$_6$
- Functions
  - Coenzyme in protein and amino acid metabolism
  - Supports immune system
- Food sources
  - Meat, fish, poultry, liver
  - Potatoes, bananas, watermelon, sunflower seeds
- Deficiency
  - Microcytic hypochromic anemia
- Toxicity
  - Can cause permanent nerve damage in high doses

Folate
- Functions
  - Coenzyme in DNA synthesis and cell division
  - Needed for normal red blood cell synthesis
- Food sources
  - Green leafy vegetables, orange juice, legumes
  - Fortified cereals, enriched grains
- Deficiency
  - Megaloblastic anemia
  - Can contribute to neural tube defects
  - All women need 400 micrograms/day of folic acid
- Toxicity
  - Can mask vitamin B$_{12}$ deficiency

Vitamin B$_{12}$
- Functions
  - Needed for normal folate function
    - DNA and red blood cell synthesis
  - Maintains myelin sheath around nerves
- Food sources
  - Only animal foods: meats, liver, milk, eggs
- Deficiency
  - Pernicious anemia
    - Megaloblastic anemia + nerve damage

Notes

Pantothenic Acid and Biotin

- Functions of pantothenic acid
  - Component of Coenzyme A
- Food sources of pantothenic acid
  - Widespread in foods
- Functions of biotin
  - Amino acid metabolism
  - Fatty acid synthesis
  - DNA synthesis
- Food sources of biotin
  - Cauliflower, liver, peanuts, cheese

Vitamin C

- Functions
  - Antioxidant
  - Needed for collagen synthesis
- Food sources
  - Fruits: citrus, strawberries, kiwi
  - Vegetables: broccoli, tomatoes, potatoes
- Deficiency
  - Scurvy
- Toxicity
  - May cause GI distress in high doses

Spotlight on Alcohol

Notes

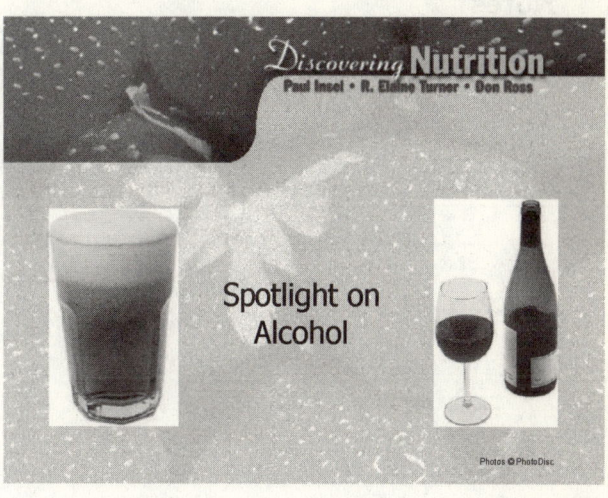

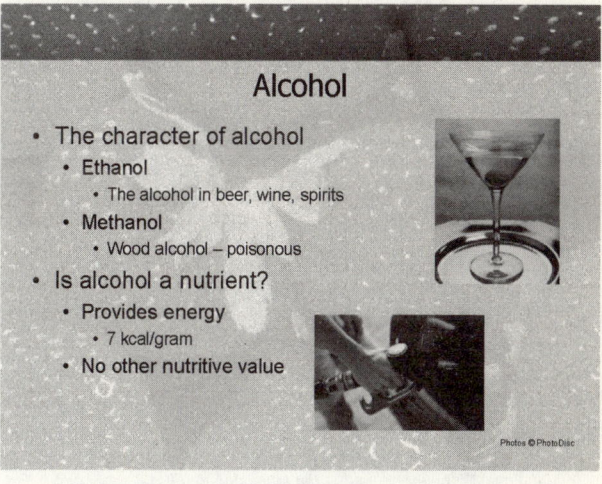

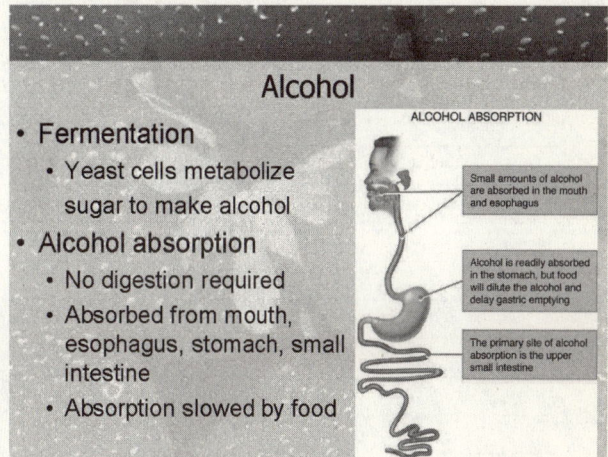

Notes

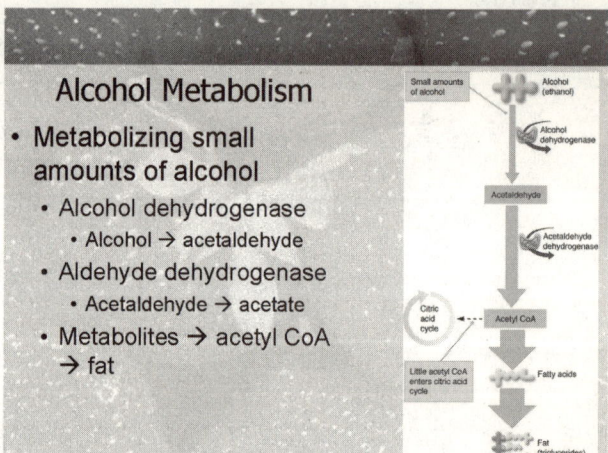

Alcohol Metabolism
- **Metabolizing small amounts of alcohol**
  - Alcohol dehydrogenase
    - Alcohol → acetaldehyde
  - Aldehyde dehydrogenase
    - Acetaldehyde → acetate
  - Metabolites → acetyl CoA → fat

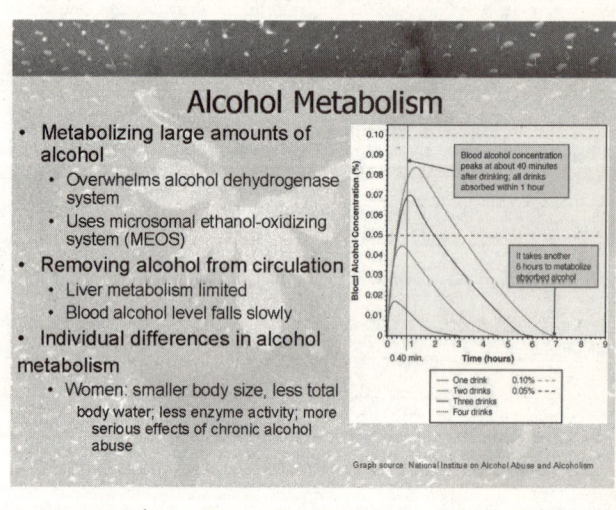

Alcohol Metabolism
- **Metabolizing large amounts of alcohol**
  - Overwhelms alcohol dehydrogenase system
  - Uses microsomal ethanol-oxidizing system (MEOS)
- **Removing alcohol from circulation**
  - Liver metabolism limited
  - Blood alcohol level falls slowly
- **Individual differences in alcohol metabolism**
  - Women: smaller body size, less total body water; less enzyme activity; more serious effects of chronic alcohol abuse

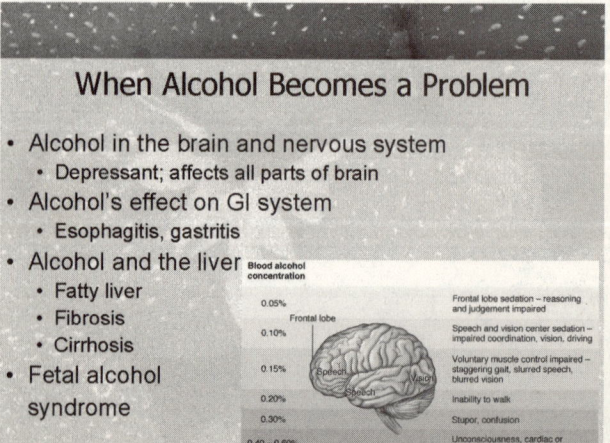

When Alcohol Becomes a Problem
- Alcohol in the brain and nervous system
  - Depressant; affects all parts of brain
- Alcohol's effect on GI system
  - Esophagitis, gastritis
- Alcohol and the liver
  - Fatty liver
  - Fibrosis
  - Cirrhosis
- Fetal alcohol syndrome

Alcoholics and Malnutrition

- Poor diet
  - Alcohol – energy but no nutrients
  - Economic factors
  - Lack of interest in food; GI problems
- Vitamin deficiencies
  - Alcohol interferes with vitamin metabolism
  - Folate, thiamin, vitamin A

Alcoholics and Malnutrition

- Mineral deficiencies
  - Inadequate diet and fluid losses
  - Calcium, magnesium, iron, zinc
  - Some mineral levels are elevated
- Macronutrients
  - Alcohol interferes with amino acid absorption
  - Alcohol raises blood levels of fats
- Body weight
  - Inconsistent effect of alcohol calories on weight

Does Alcohol Have Benefits?

- Moderate drinking associated with reduced mortality
- Heart disease
  - French paradox: red wine

Notes

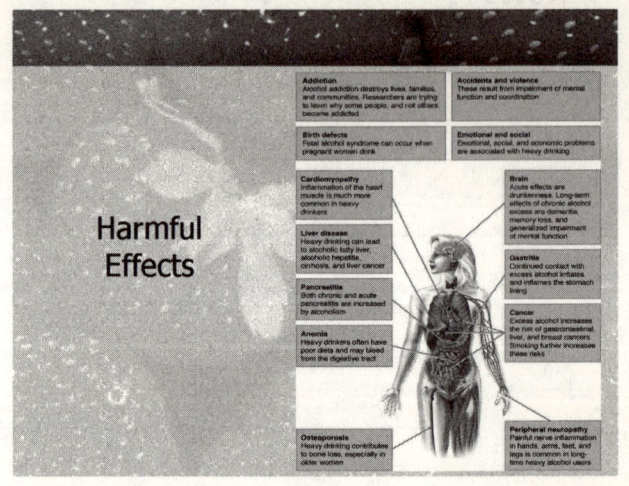

Chapter 10: Water and Minerals: The Ocean Within

Notes

Water and Minerals: The Ocean Within

Water: Crucial to Life

- **Functions**
  - Moves nutrients and wastes
  - Lubricates joints
  - Participates in chemical reactions
  - Helps maintain body temperature
- **Water needs**
  - 1-1.5 milliters per kilocalorie
- **Water balance**
  - Intake vs. excretion
  - Dehydration

Major Minerals and Health

- **Hypertension: high blood pressure**
  - Increases risk for heart disease, stroke, kidney disease
  - Sodium
    - Can increase blood pressure in some people
  - Other dietary factors
    - Increase BP: chloride
    - Decrease BP: calcium, magnesium, potassium

Notes

Major Minerals and Health

- Osteoporosis
  - Decreased bone density
  - Develops gradually with age
  - Women at higher risk
  - Factors to reduce risk
    - Adequate calcium intake throughout life
    - Regular exercise

Sodium

- Functions
  - Fluid balance
  - Nerve impulse transmission
- Food sources and recommended intake
  - Salt
  - Processed and convenience foods
  - Limit to 2,400 milligrams/day (DV)

Potassium and Chloride

- Functions of potassium
  - Muscle contraction
  - Nerve impulse transmission
  - Fluid balance
- Food sources of potassium
  - Unprocessed foods: fruits, vegetables, grains
- Functions of chloride
  - Fluid balance
  - Hydrochloric acid (stomach acid)
- Food sources of chloride
  - Table salt

Calcium

- Functions
  - Bone structure
  - Blood clotting
  - Nerve impulse transmission, muscle contraction
- Food sources
  - Milk and dairy products
  - Green vegetables, tofu, fortified foods
- Calcium absorption
  - Reduced by fiber, phytates, oxalates
- Calcium balance
  - Lack of calcium can contribute to osteoporosis

Phosphorus and Magnesium

- Functions of phosphorus
  - Bone structure
  - Component of ATP, DNA, RNA, phospholipids
- Food sources of phosphorus
  - Meat, milk, eggs
  - Processed foods
- Functions
  - DNA and protein synthesis
  - Blood clotting, muscle contraction, ATP production
- Food sources
  - Whole grains, vegetables, legumes, tofu, seafood

Iron

- Functions
  - Oxygen transport as part of hemoglobin and myoglobin
  - Cofactor for enzymes, normal brain and immune function
- Food sources
  - Red meats, liver, seafood
- Deficiency
  - Iron-deficiency anemia
- Toxicity
  - Poisoning in children
  - Hemochromatosis

Water and Minerals: The Ocean Within

Notes

Zinc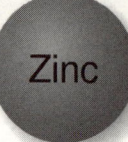

- Functions
  - Cofactor for enzymes
  - Gene regulation, immune health
- Food sources
  - Red meats, seafood
- Deficiency
  - Poor growth, delayed development
- Toxicity
  - Can cause copper deficiency

Selenium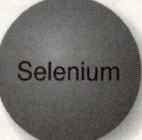

- Functions
  - Part of antioxidant enzyme
  - Thyroid metabolism, immune function
- Food sources
  - Organ meats, fish, seafood, meats, Brazil nuts
- Deficiency
  - Increases susceptibility to some infections
- Toxicity
  - Brittle hair and nails

Iodine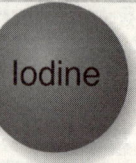

- Functions
  - Thyroid hormone production
- Food sources
  - Iodized salt, fish, seafood, dairy products
- Deficiency
  - Goiter: enlarged thyroid gland
  - Cretinism: mental retardation
    - Occurs in fetus when pregnant woman is deficient

Notes

Copper and Manganese

- **Functions of copper**
  - Melanin, collagen, elastin production
  - Immune function
  - Antioxidant enzyme systems
- **Food sources of copper**
  - Organ meats, shellfish, nuts, legumes
- **Functions of manganese**
  - Cartilage production
  - Antioxidant enzyme systems
- **Food sources of manganese**
  - Tea, coffee, nuts, cereals

Fluoride and Chromium

- **Functions of fluoride**
  - Bone and tooth structure
- **Food sources of fluoride**
  - Fluoridated water
- **Fluoride balance**
  - Excess can cause fluorosis
- **Functions of chromium**
  - Glucose metabolism
- **Food sources of chromium**
  - Mushrooms, dark chocolate, nuts, whole grains

Chapter 11: Sports Nutrition: Eating for Peak Performance

Notes

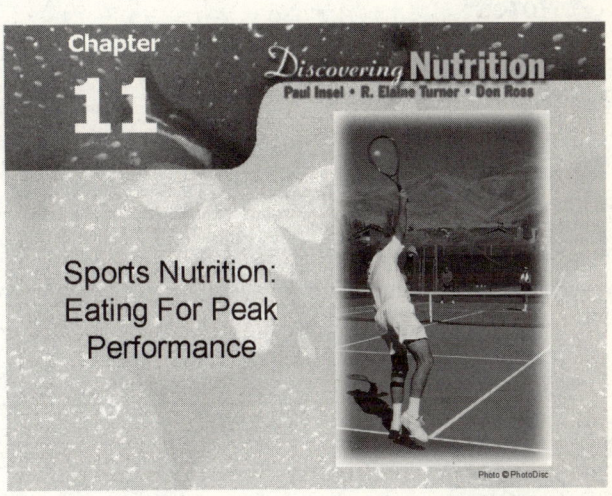

Sports Nutrition: Eating For Peak Performance

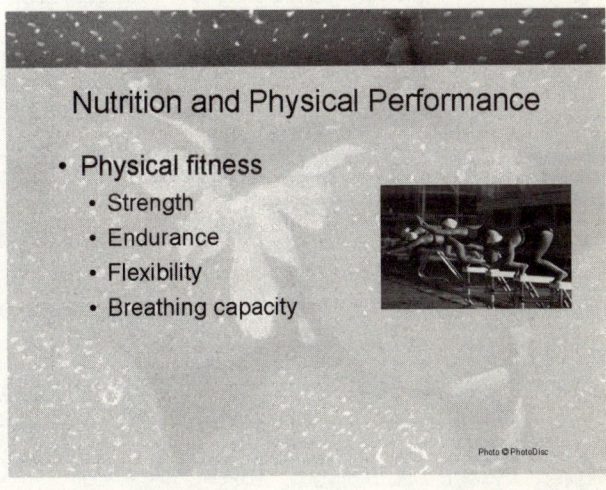

Nutrition and Physical Performance

- Physical fitness
  - Strength
  - Endurance
  - Flexibility
  - Breathing capacity

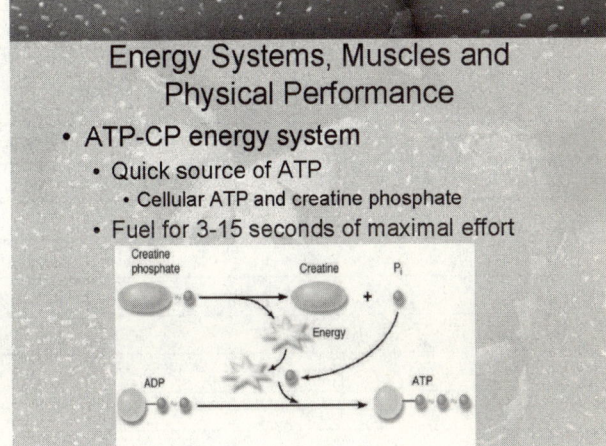

Energy Systems, Muscles and Physical Performance

- ATP-CP energy system
  - Quick source of ATP
    - Cellular ATP and creatine phosphate
  - Fuel for 3-15 seconds of maximal effort

Notes

Energy Systems, Muscles and Physical Performance

- **Lactic acid energy system**
  - Breakdown of glucose to lactic acid (lactate)
    - Doesn't require oxygen
  - Rise in acidity triggers muscle fatigue

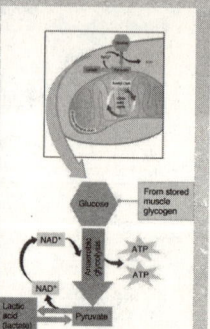

Energy Systems, Muscles and Physical Performance

- **Oxygen energy system**
  - Breakdown of carbohydrate and fat for energy
    - Requires oxygen
    - Produces ATP more slowly

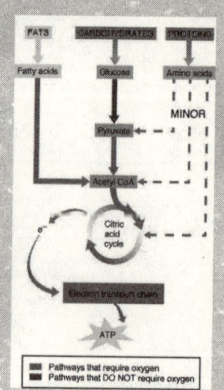

Energy Systems, Muscles, and Physical Performance

- Teamwork in energy production
  - Anaerobic systems for short duration activities, early part of endurance activities
  - Aerobic systems for endurance activities
- Glycogen depletion
  - Limited stores of glycogen
- Training
  - Decreases reliance on anaerobic systems
  - Extends availability of glycogen

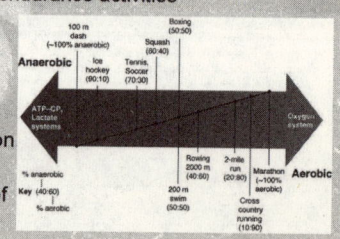

Optimal Nutrition for Athletic Performance

- General recommendations
  - Consume adequate energy and nutrients to support health and performance
  - Maintain appropriate body composition
  - Promote optimal recovery from training
  - Maintain hydration status

Carbohydrate and Exercise

- High carbohydrate diets
  - Increase glycogen stores
  - Extend endurance
- Carbohydrate loading
- Carbohydrates intake
  - Before exercise: 2-4 hours before
  - During exercise: beverages
  - After exercise: 1-1.5 grams/kg weight 30 minutes and 2 hours after

Fat and Exercise

- Fat
  - Major fuel source for endurance activities
  - High fat diet not needed
  - Recommendations
    - Moderate fat intake < 30% of calories

Notes

Protein and Exercise

- Protein recommendations
  - Adults: 0.8 grams/kg body weight
  - Endurance athletes: 1.2-1.4 grams/kg
  - Strength athletes: 1.6-1.7 grams/kg
- Protein sources
  - Foods: lean meats, fish, low-fat dairy, egg whites
- Protein intake after exercise
  - Helps replenish glycogen
- Dangers of high protein intake

Vitamins, Minerals, and Athletic Performance

- B vitamins
  - Needed for energy metabolism
  - Choose variety of whole grains, fruits, vegetables
- Calcium
  - Needed for normal muscle function, strong bones
  - Low-fat dairy products
  - Adequate intake may be a problem for females
- Iron
  - Needed for oxygen delivery and energy production
  - Athletes have higher losses
  - Lean red meats, vegetables, enriched grains

Fluid Needs During Exercise

- **Exercise and fluid loss**
  - Increased losses from sweat
  - Increased with heat, humidity
  - Risk for dehydration
- **Hydration**
  - Adequate fluids before, during, after exercise
  - Water vs. sports drinks

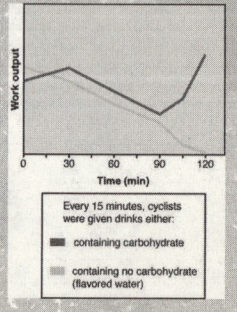

Every 15 minutes, cyclists were given drinks either:
- containing carbohydrate
- containing no carbohydrate (flavored water)

Notes

Nutrition Supplements and Ergogenic Aids

- Many product claims
  - Energy, enhance performance, change body composition
  - Limited scientific evidence
  - Potential for side effects
  - Many substances are banned for athletes
- Popular supplements

Weight and Body Composition

- Weight gain
  - Increase muscle, reduce fat
- Weight loss
  - Lose fat, maintain muscle
  - Dangerous weight loss practices
- Female athlete triad
  - Disordered eating
  - Amenorrhea
  - Osteoporosis

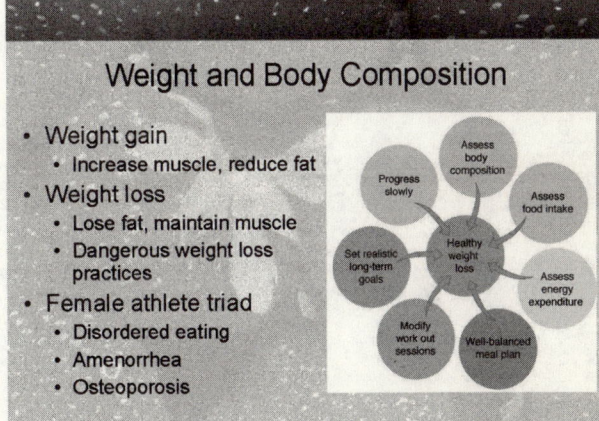

Spotlight on Eating Disorders

Notes

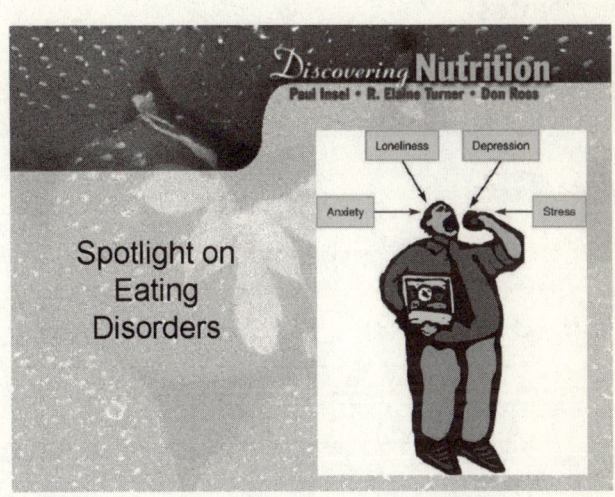

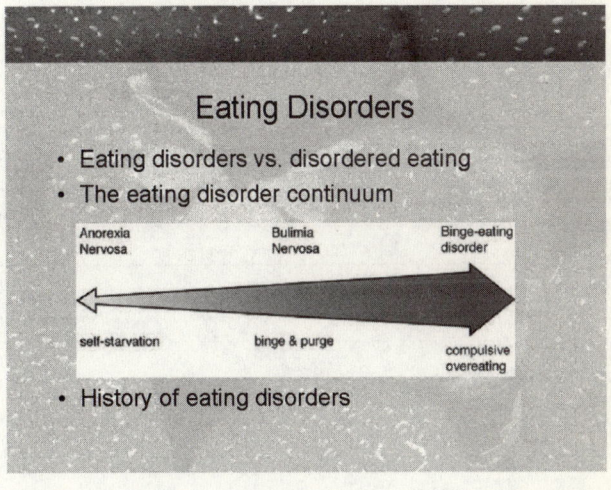

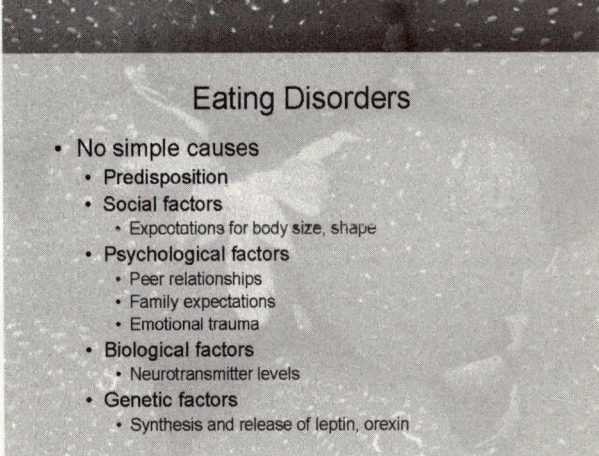

Notes

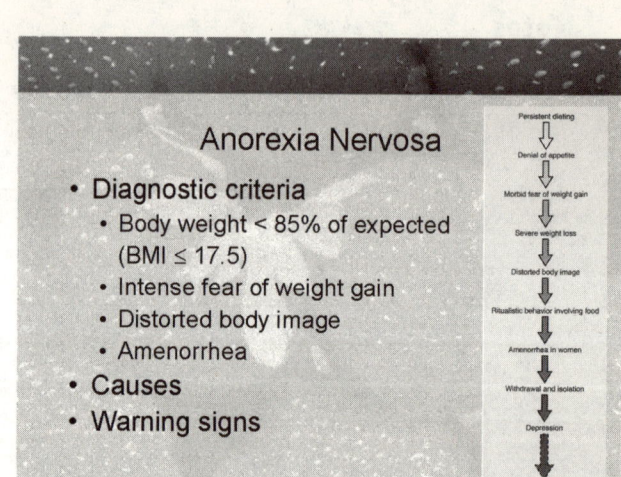

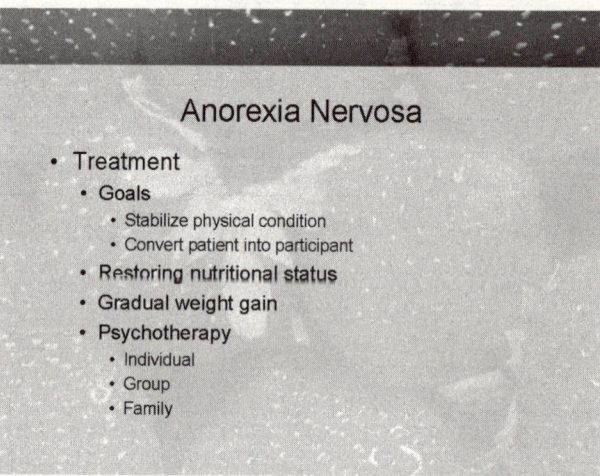

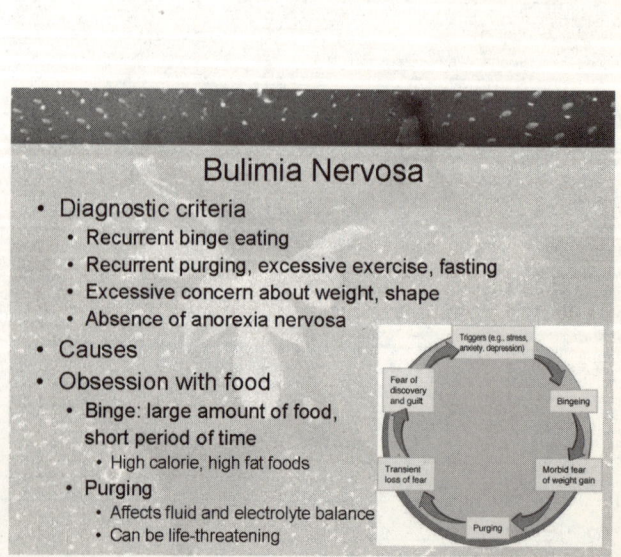

Notes

Bulimia Nervosa

- Treatment
  - Medical
  - Nutritional
  - Psychotherapy
    - Antidepressant medications

Binge-Eating Disorder

- Diagnostic criteria
  - Recurrent binge eating
  - Distress over eating behaviors
  - No recurrent purging
  - Absence of anorexia nervosa
- Triggers of binge eating
  - Stress
  - Conflict
  - Frequent dieting

Binge-Eating Disorder

- Treatment
  - Psychotherapy
    - Antidepressant medications
  - Long-term support

Spotlight on Eating Disorders

Notes

Eating Disorders

- Males: an overlooked population
  - Fewer instances than females
  - Men involved in sports, modeling, entertainment
    - Pressure for certain weight, shape
- Anorexia athletica
  - Sports-related eating disorders
  - Body size/shape important in competition
  - Pressure from coaches

Eating Disorders

- **Female athlete triad**
  - Disordered eating
  - Amenorrhea
  - Osteoporosis
- **Vegetarianism and eating disorders**
- **Smoking and eating disorders**
- **Baryophobia**
- **Infantile anorexia**

Eating Disorders

- **Combating eating disorders**
  - Promote self-esteem
  - Size acceptance

Chapter 12: Life Cycle: Maternal and Infant Nutrition

Notes

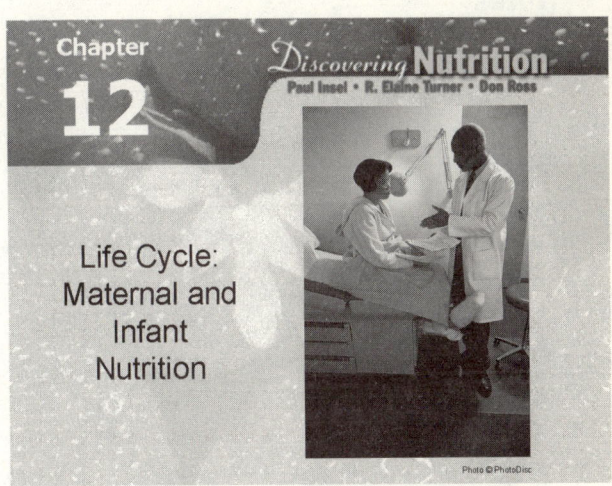

Pregnancy

- Nutrition before conception
  - Risk assessment, health promotion, intervention
  - Weight
    - Maintain a healthy weight
  - Vitamins
    - 400 micrograms folic acid/day
    - Avoid high doses of vitamin A (retinol)
  - Substance use
    - Eliminate prior to pregnancy

Pregnancy

- Physiology of pregnancy
  - Stages of human fetal growth
    - Blastogenic stage: first 2 weeks
      - Cells differentiate into fetus, placenta
    - Embryonic stage: weeks 2-8
      - Development of organ systems
    - Fetal stage: week 9-delivery
      - Growth

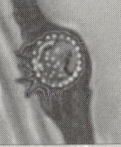
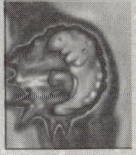

Notes

Pregnancy

- Physiology of pregnancy
  - Maternal physiological changes
    - Growth of adipose, breast, uterine tissues
    - Increase blood volume
    - Slower GI motility

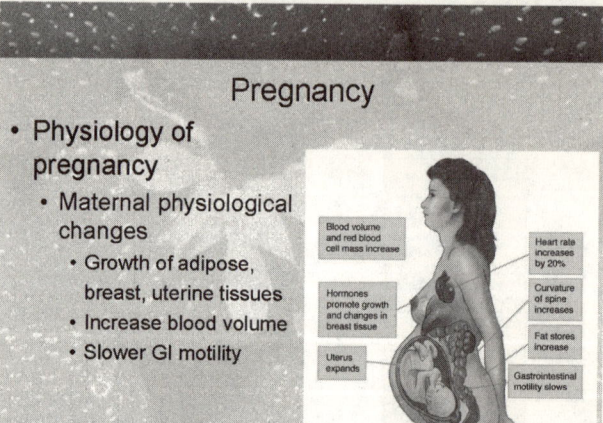

Pregnancy

- Maternal weight gain
  - Recommendations depend on BMI
    - Normal weight (BMI = 19.8 – 26)
      - Gain 25-35 pounds
- Energy and nutrition during pregnancy
  - Energy
    - Support adequate weight gain
  - Macronutrients
    - High carbohydrate, moderate fat and protein

Pregnancy

- Energy and nutrition during pregnancy
  - Micronutrients
    - Increase need for most vitamins and minerals
    - Highest increase for iron and folate
- Food choices for pregnant women
  - Pyramid-style diet
  - Supplements of iron and folate
- Substance use
  - Risk for birth defects, low birth weight, preterm delivery

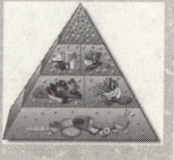

Notes

Pregnancy

- Special situations
  - Gastrointestinal distress
  - Food cravings and aversions
  - Hypertension
  - Diabetes
  - Gestational diabetes
  - AIDS
  - Adolescence

Lactation

- Physiology of lactation
- Changes during pregnancy
  - Increased breast tissue
  - Maturation of structure
- Hormonal controls
  - Prolactin: stimulates milk production
  - Oxytocin: stimulates milk release
    - "let-down" reflex

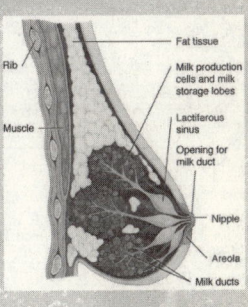

Lactation

- Nutrition for breastfeeding women
  - Energy and protein
    - higher needs than pregnancy
  - Vitamins and minerals
    - Most are higher or same as pregnancy
    - Iron and folate needs are lower
  - Water
- Food choices
- Practices to avoid while breastfeeding
  - Alcohol, drugs, smoking, excess caffeine

Life Cycle: Maternal and Infant Nutrition

Notes

Lactation
- Benefits of breastfeeding
  - Benefits for infants
    - Optimal nutrition
    - Reduced incidence of respiratory, GI, ear infections
    - Convenience
    - Other benefits
  - Benefits for mother
    - Convenience
    - Enhance recovery of uterus size
    - Other benefits
- Contraindications to breastfeeding

Infancy
- Infant growth and development
  - Growth best marker of nutritional status
    - Evaluated using growth charts
  - Weight gain
    - Double birth weight by 4-6 months
    - Triple birth weight by 12 months
  - Length gain
    - Increase length by 50% by 12 months
  - Head circumference

Infancy
- Energy and nutrient needs of infancy
  - Requirements based on composition of breast milk
  - Energy
    - Highest needs of any life stage
      - ~ 100 kcals/kg/day
  - Protein
    - Highest needs of any life stage
      - ~ 2 g/kg/day
  - Carbohydrate and fat
    - Fat major energy source
    - Carbohydrates as simple sugars
  - Water

Protein
Growth

Carbohydrate (lactose)
Energy
Enhances absorption of calcium and phosphorus

Fat
Energy
Nervous system development
Accumulation of fat stores

Notes

Infancy

- **Energy and nutrient needs of infancy**
  - Key vitamins and minerals
    - Vitamin D
    - Vitamin K
    - Vitamin B12
    - Iron
    - Fluoride
  - Feeding infants
    - Breastfeeding
    - Infant formula

Infancy

- **Introduction of solid foods**
  - Readiness for solids
    - Increased digestive enzymes
    - Loss of extrusion reflex
    - Able to sit without support
    - Age of about 4-6 months
  - Feeding schedule
    - Baby rice cereal
    - Strained fruits, vegetables, meats
    - Add one food at a time

Infancy

- **Feeding problems during infancy**
  - Colic
  - Baby bottle tooth decay
  - Iron-deficiency anemia
  - Gastroesophageal reflux
  - Diarrhea
  - Failure to thrive

Life Cycle: Maternal and Infant Nutrition

Chapter 13: Life Cycle: From Childhood through Adulthood

Notes

Life Cycle: From Childhood through Adulthood

Childhood

- Energy and nutrient needs during childhood
  - Energy and protein
    - Kcal and grams protein per kg decrease from infancy
  - Vitamins and minerals
    - Variety of foods needed
    - Need for supplements?
- Influences on childhood food habits and intake

Childhood

- Nutritional concerns of childhood
  - Malnutrition and hunger
    - School Lunch, Breakfast, and Summer Food Service programs
  - Food and behavior
    - No scientific link between diet and hyperactivity
  - Nutrition and chronic disease
    - Gradually phase in lower-fat, higher-fiber diet
  - Childhood obesity
    - Increasing incidence
    - Focus on growth
  - Lead toxicity
  - Vegetarianism

Notes

Adolescence

- Physical growth and development
  - Adolescent growth spurt
    - Boys: begins between 12-13 years
      - Gain about 8 inches in height, 45 pounds in weight
    - Girls: begins between 10-11 years
      - Gain about 6 inches in height, 35 pounds in weight
  - Change in body composition
  - Changes in emotional maturity

Adolescence

- Nutrient needs of adolescents
  - Energy and protein
    - Highest total calories and protein grams per day
  - Vitamins and minerals of concern
    - Vitamin A
    - Iron
    - Calcium
- Influences on food intake
  - Social factors
  - Income
  - Individuality

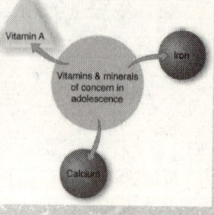

Adolescence

- Nutrition-related concerns of adolescents
  - Fitness and sports
  - Acne
  - Eating disorders
  - Obesity
  - Tobacco, alcohol, recreational drugs

Notes

Staying Young While Growing Older

- Age-related changes
  - Weight and body composition
    - Add fat, lose lean body mass
  - Mobility
    - Reduced muscle and skeletal strength
  - Immunity
    - Decline in defense mechanism
  - Taste and smell
    - Decline in ability
  - Gastrointestinal changes
    - Reduced acid secretion, reduced motility

Nutrient Needs of the Mature Adult

- Energy
  - Reduced needs
    - Decreased activity, decreased lean body mass
- Protein
  - Same needs per kg body weight as younger adults
- Carbohydrate
  - More likely to be lactose intolerant
- Fat
  - Maintain moderate-low fat diet
- Water
  - Reduced thirst response

Nutrient Needs of the Mature Adult

- Vitamins of concern
  - Vitamin D
    - Needed for bone health, calcium balance
    - Reduced skin synthesis, activation
    - Higher needs
  - B vitamins
    - Reduced ability to absorb vitamin B_{12}
    - Folate, B_6, B_{12} may help reduce heart disease risk

Notes

Nutrient Needs of the Mature Adult

- Minerals of concern
  - Calcium
    - Bone health
    - Reduced ability to absorb calcium
  - Zinc
    - Marginal deficiencies likely
    - May compromise immunity, wound healing
  - Magnesium
  - Iron
    - Elders may have limited intake
- Need for supplements

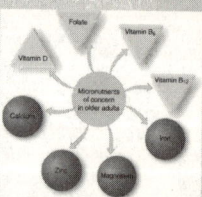

Nutrition-Related Concerns of Mature Adults

- Drug-drug and drug-nutrient interactions
  - Can affect use of drugs or nutrients
- Depression
  - May reduce food intake
  - Alcoholism can interfere with nutrient use
- Anorexia of aging
  - Loss of appetite with illness
  - Can lead to protein-energy malnutrition

Nutrition-Related Concerns of Mature Adults

- Arthritis
  - May interfere with food preparation and eating
  - Dietary changes may improve symptoms
- Bowel and bladder regulation
  - Increased risk of urinary tract infection
  - Chronic constipation more common with age
    - Need for increased fluids, fiber
- Dental health
  - May interfere with eating ability, food choices

Notes

Nutrition-Related Concerns of Mature Adults

- Vision problems
    - Can affect ability to shop, cook
    - Antioxidants may reduce macular degeneration
- Osteoporosis
    - Common in elders, especially women
    - Maintain calcium, vitamin D, exercise
- Alzheimer's disease
    - Affects ability to function
    - Reduced taste, smell
    - Risk for weight loss, malnutrition

Meal Management for Mature Adults

- **Managing independently**
    - Services for elders
        - Meals on Wheels
        - Elderly Nutrition Program
        - Food Stamp Program
- **Wise eating for one or two**
- **Finding community resources**

Chapter 14: Food Safety and Technology: Microbial Threats and Genetic Engineering

Notes

Food Safety and Technology

- Microbial Threats and Genetic Engineering

Food Safety

- Harmful substances in foods
  - Pathogens
    - Bacteria, viruses, parasites
  - Foodborne illness
    - Infection from pathogen
    - Toxin produced by microorganism
  - Common causes of foodborne illness
    - *Staphylococcus aureus*
    - *Clostridium botulinum*
    - *Salmonella*
    - *Escherichia coli*

Food Safety

- Harmful substances in food
  - Chemical contamination
    - Pesticides
      - Organic alternatives
    - Animal drugs
    - Pollutants
  - Natural toxins
    - Aflatoxins
    - Ciguatera
    - Methyl mercury
    - Poisonous mushrooms
    - Solanine
  - Other food contaminants

Notes

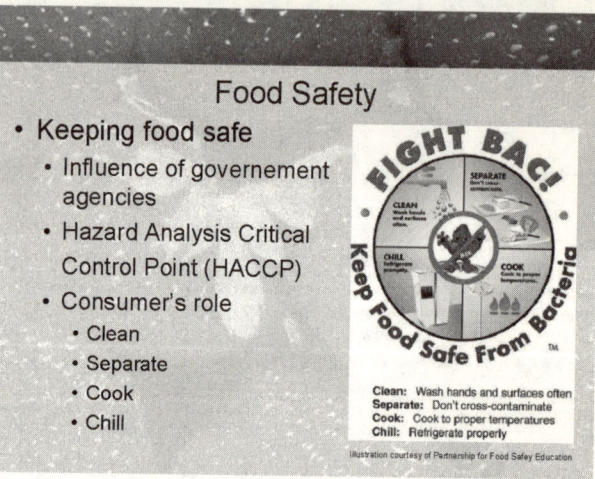

Food Safety
- Keeping food safe
  - Influence of governement agencies
  - Hazard Analysis Critical Control Point (HACCP)
  - Consumer's role
    - Clean
    - Separate
    - Cook
    - Chill

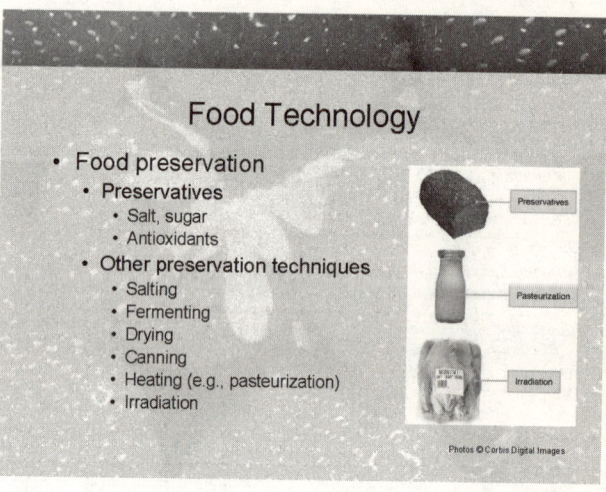

Food Technology
- Food preservation
  - Preservatives
    - Salt, sugar
    - Antioxidants
  - Other preservation techniques
    - Salting
    - Fermenting
    - Drying
    - Canning
    - Heating (e.g., pasteurization)
    - Irradiation

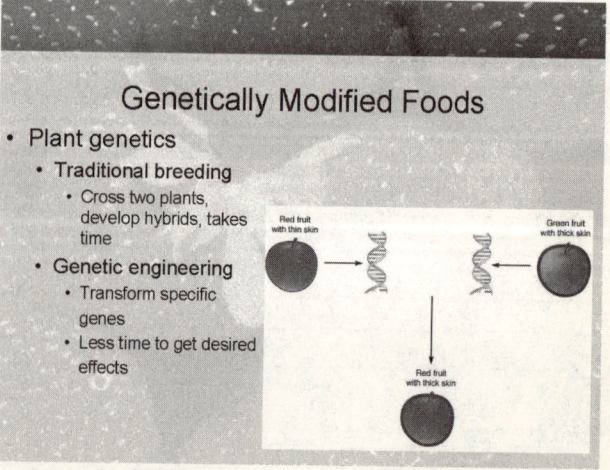

Genetically Modified Foods
- Plant genetics
  - Traditional breeding
    - Cross two plants, develop hybrids, takes time
  - Genetic engineering
    - Transform specific genes
    - Less time to get desired effects

Notes

Genetically Modified Foods

- Benefits of genetic engineering
  - Enhanced plant growth
  - Reduced pesticide, fertilizer use
  - Enhanced nutrient composition
  - Enhanced crop yields
- Risks
  - Potential for new allergens
  - Herbicide resistant weeds
  - Loss of biodiversity

Genetically Modified Foods

- Regulation
  - FDA oversees GM foods
  - Label requirements
    - If food is significantly different
    - If there are issues regarding use of the food
    - If food has different nutritional properties
    - If new food contains unexpected allergen

Chapter 15: World View of Nutrition: The Faces of Global Malnutrition

Notes

World View of Nutrition
The Faces of Global Malnutrition

Malnutrition in the United States

- Food insecurity
  - Anxiety about having enough to eat
  - Worry about having no money to buy food
- Prevalence and distribution
  - Strongly associated with poverty
  - Linked with economic and social factors

Malnutrition in the United States

- Groups at risk for hunger and malnutrition
  - The working poor
    - May or may not qualify for food assistance
  - The isolated
    - Lack access to food resources
  - Elders
    - Economic difficulties
    - Physical ailments

Notes

Malnutrition in the United States

- Groups at risk for hunger and malnutrition
  - The homeless
    - Lack consistent cooking facilities
    - Limited income, if any
  - Children
    - Dependent on family circumstances
    - Hunger affects school performance

Malnutrition in the United States

- Attacking hunger in America
  - The Food Stamp program
    - Extends food buying power
  - Special Supplemental Nutrition Program for Women, Infants, and Children (WIC)
    - Food, nutrition services for pregnant and lactating women, and children to age 5
  - National School Lunch Program
    - Free and reduced price meals
  - Child and Adult Care Food Program

Malnutrition in the Developing World

- Factors that contribute to hunger and malnutrition
  - Social and economic factors
    - Poverty
    - Population growth
    - Urbanization
  - Infection and disease

Notes

Malnutrition in the Developing World

- Factors that contribute to hunger and malnutrition
  - Political disruptions and natural disasters
    - War
    - Refugees
    - Sanctions
    - Floods, droughts, mudslides, hurricanes
  - Inequitable food distribution

Malnutrition in the Developing World

- Agriculture and environment: a tricky balance
  - Environmental degradation
    - Reduced food production
    - Nutritional consequences

Malnutrition in the Developing World

- Common forms of malnutrition
  - Protein-energy malnutrition
    - Kwashiorkor
    - Marasmus
    - Breastfeeding often key to child's survival
  - Iodine deficiency disorders
    - Most common cause of preventable brain damage

Notes

Malnutrition in the Developing World

- Common forms of malnutrition
  - Vitamin A deficiency
    - Leading cause of preventable blindness
  - Iron-deficiency anemia
    - Limits productive of population
  - Other vitamin, mineral deficiencies
  - Overweight and obesity
    - Differing cultural attitudes
    - High calorie, low nutrient dense foods

Notes

Notes

Notes

Notes

Notes

Notes

Notes

Notes

Notes

Notes